JAMES KENT, PsyD
RONNIE KENT, MD

the Anxiety ALGORITHM

◇◇◇

TURNING YOUR PATTERN OF
WORRY AND STRESS INTO A PATTERN OF
PEACE AND JOY

Note: This book is not intended to provide medical or psychological advice or to take the place of medical advice and treatment from your personal physician. Those who are having suicidal thoughts or who have been emotionally, physically, or sexually abused should seek help from a mental health professional or qualified counselor. Neither the publisher nor the author nor the author's ministry or business takes any responsibility for any possible consequences from any action taken by any person reading or following the information in this book. If readers are taking prescription medications, they should consult with their physicians and not take themselves off prescribed medicines without the proper supervision of a physician. Always consult your physician or another qualified health care professional before undertaking any change in your physical regimen, whether fasting, diet, medications, or exercise.

Unless otherwise indicated, all Scripture quotations are taken from the *Holy Bible, New International Version*®, niv®, © 1973, 1978, 1984, 2011 by Biblica, Inc.® Used by permission. All rights reserved worldwide. The "NIV" and "New International Version" are trademarks registered in the United States Patent and Trademark Office by Biblica, Inc.® Scripture quotations marked (esv) are taken from *The Holy Bible, English Standard Version*, © 2000, 2001, 1995 by Crossway Bibles, a division of Good News Publishers. Used by permission. All rights reserved. Scripture quotations marked (tlb) are taken from *The Living Bible*, © 1971. Used by permission of Tyndale House Publishers, Inc., Carol Stream, Illinois 60188. All rights reserved. Scripture quotations marked (kjv) are taken from the King James Version of the Holy Bible. Scripture quotations marked (nlt) are taken from the *Holy Bible, New Living Translation*, © 1996, 2004, 2015 by Tyndale House Foundation. Used by permission of Tyndale House Publishers, Inc., Carol Stream, Illinois 60188. All rights reserved.

Boldface type in the Scripture quotations indicates the authors' emphasis.

James Kent, PsyD
Ronnie Kent, MD
1230Ministry.com

The Anxiety Algorithm:
Turning Your Pattern of Worry and Stress into a Pattern of Peace and Joy

ISBN: 979-8-88769-328-6
eBook ISBN: 979-8-88769-329-3
Printed in the United States of America
© 2025 by James Kent, PsyD, and Ronnie Kent, MD

Whitaker House
1030 Hunt Valley Circle
New Kensington, PA 15068
www.whitakerhouse.com

LC record available at https://lccn.loc.gov/2024036143
LC ebook record available at https://lccn.loc.gov/2024036144

No part of this book may be reproduced or transmitted in any form or by any means, electronic or mechanical—including photocopying, recording, or by any information storage and retrieval system—without permission in writing from the publisher. Please direct your inquiries to permissionseditor@whitakerhouse.com.

1 2 3 4 5 6 7 8 9 10 11 ꟽ 32 31 30 29 28 27 26 25

CONTENTS

Dedication 5
A Note to the Reader 6

PART ONE: DISCOVERING A NEW WAY TO LIVE

A Different Approach to Anxiety 9
  1. Breakthrough Moment 13
  2. What Is Wellness? 18
     Wellness Exercise: Deep Breathing 23
  3. Thinking About How We Think 25
  4. The Science of Anxiety 30
     Wellness Exercise: Progressive Muscle Relaxation ... 37
  5. Focus, Think, and Practice 40
  6. Anxiety, Fear, and the "Two Steps Back" Strategy ... 45
     Wellness Exercise: Self-Care 55
  7. Healing Broken Humans 58
  8. Moving Toward God and Wellness 68
     Wellness Exercise: Scripture Visualization 76
  9. Giving Ourselves to God 80
 10. Unpacking Our Strength and Mind 85
 11. Unpacking Our Soul and Heart 91
     Wellness Exercise: Scripture Memorization 100

PART TWO: APPLYING THE ANXIETY ALGORITHM

12. The Algorithm Plan 105
13. Personalizing the Algorithm 112
14. Creating New Pathways 120
    Wellness Exercise: A Daily Quiet Time 127
15. Mapping the Journey 129
    Wellness Exercise: The Thought Record Method 143

PART THREE: OVERCOMING ANXIETY THROUGH STRONG RELATIONSHIPS

16. Building Strong Relationships, Part 1 153
    Wellness Exercise: Genogram and Spiritual Timeline 164
17. Building Strong Relationships, Part 2 166
    Wellness Exercise: Make Gratitude Your Attitude! 174
18. Reducing Anxiety Through Effective Communication 176
    Wellness Exercise: Good Communication Techniques 189

PART FOUR: THE ALGORITHM AND LONG-TERM WELLNESS

19. A Life of Wellness 193
20. Discovering True Joy 208
    Wellness Exercise: Engage in Spiritual Practices 220
21. The Algorithm and Prayer 222
    Wellness Exercise: Pray the Names of God 239
22. The Secret of Contentment 240

An Invitation 246
Examples of Personalizing the Anxiety Algorithm 249
Acknowledgments 254
About the Authors 255

To Anne, the love of my life and my partner on this journey: you inspire me to the task.

To my children Emily, James, and Grace (the three your mother and I welcomed through birth) and Troy, Jessica, and Casey (the three we welcomed through marriage): you encourage me greatly by your parenting skills, and you give me great hope for the future.

To my ten grandchildren, Mary Brooke, Caleb, Covington, Winston, Wylder, Hudson, Eve, Roman, Kent, and Ellie: you make me so happy to get up every morning.

> *"I have no greater joy than to hear that my children are walking in the truth."* (3 John 4)

—RONNIE

To Jessica, my wife, and my children.

To all those who are looking for peace: may you come to know the God of peace and experience His unfailing presence.

—JAMES

A NOTE TO THE READER

In writing this book, both of us (James Kent and Ronnie Kent) agreed that we would use the term "we" when speaking of our shared perspectives, theology, and practices. We also agreed that any time one of us was speaking of our unique experiences and contributions, we would use the term "I" followed by one of our names in parentheses: (James) or (Ronnie).

We both affirm that our theological and clinic approaches to anxiety are essentially the same and that we are learning from each other in order to better live out and teach what it means to have a life established in the peace of Christ and to experience the fullness of life He promises.

Part One:

DISCOVERING A NEW WAY TO LIVE

A DIFFERENT APPROACH TO ANXIETY

I (Ronnie) worked in pediatrics for forty-one years, and I'll never forget when I was called to the emergency room to see a twelve-year-old boy named Shane who had a bump on his head. I had just started my practice in Hattiesburg, Mississippi. Although I was fresh out of my residency, as a pediatrician, I had already seen a lot of bumps on the head. Kids are resilient, and their bodies are flexible and able to withstand tumbles and falls that would be downright dangerous for adults. At the same time, kids are kids. They fall, flop, and drop like it's their life calling, and so it wasn't out of the ordinary for parents to bring their child to the ER following a particularly scary fall. Most of the time, the child's injuries weren't serious, and I sent the family on their way, assuring them that everything would be fine.

When I went into the exam room, this situation looked no different. There sat a bright-eyed, alert young boy and a relatively calm mother. I felt I would be able to do what I usually did—take a brief history, do a neurological exam, reassure the mother, and send them home.

But then I asked a routine question that changed everything—it changed that day, it changed my relationship with that twelve-year-old boy, and, to be honest, it changed my life. I asked his mother, "Does he have any other health problems?"

"Shane has hemophilia."

That statement turned the boy's supposedly short ER visit into a prolonged stay in the intensive care unit, where he needed to have CT scans and be given medication intravenously.

Shane needed help because, due to his hemophilia, his blood couldn't clot on its own. He was at risk of having a fatal cerebral hemorrhage, a bleed in his brain. We began to give him factor VIII, which is a blood product that is collected from many people. It helps the blood clot, thus saving the patient's life. Shane had been given factor VIII many times prior to this incident when he had previously bled, primarily in his joints.

Shane recovered from that fall, but, over the years, he needed additional transfusions of factor VIII. I continued to follow his progress. Unfortunately, as was the case for many patients with hemophilia in that era, at some point along the way, he received a transfusion or transfusions that forever changed his medical condition and his life. Unbeknownst to us, some of the factor VIII that he was given was HIV positive. Back then, we in the medical field were just discovering the HIV virus and how it is transmitted. New tests for HIV became available, and we began to screen anyone who had received a transfusion, and Shane tested positive when he was sixteen. Not only that, but one or more of the transfusions he received over the years was tainted with hepatitis C. So, Shane not only became HIV positive but also ended up contracting hepatitis C, later developing cirrhosis of the liver as a result, which almost killed him.

That was the way my journey with Shane began. All because of one bump on the head.

Shane has now been HIV positive for thirty-two years—a total miracle. He is married, is a father, and, years ago, with an IV in his arm because he was in the middle of therapy at the time, he was ordained as a pastor. He pastored Christ United Methodist Church in Memphis until he retired a few years ago to focus on a new ministry calling. Shane has lived a great life, but, throughout it, he has experienced one health crisis after another. If it wasn't directly due to the hemophilia, HIV, or hepatitis, it was clogged arteries, keratoconus (an eye disease that affects the shape of the cornea, resulting in vision loss), diabetes, and more. Despite this, he's the happiest, most Jesus-loving guy you'll ever meet. I always assumed that Shane's happiness, peace, and joy were the few things that were untouchable in his life and couldn't be shaken. But when we reconnected a few years ago, after life had taken us in separate directions for a while, I found out I was wrong.

All the success Shane had experienced as a preacher had come with a lot of expectations and pressures, and he had developed significant anxiety and panic attacks. These resulted in numerous physical symptoms, such as nausea. Before preaching, the anxiety and nausea were so bad that he would vomit, and if he had to preach a second time that day, he'd vomit again in between services. His mental peace was failing him just as his body had been failing him, and Shane was running out of options. He was on anti-anxiety medicine, and he was seeing a counselor and doing all the right things, yet he couldn't sleep at night, couldn't perform at his best. His joy and peace were gone.

After hearing about his struggle, I had a few ideas. Gleaning from the book of Philippians, I instructed Shane to approach his relationship with God and his relationship with his anxiety and depression in a different way from what he had been doing.

Shane did exactly what I said, and, before we knew it, he was sleeping through the night and no longer needed his anxiety medication. His fears and concerns no longer consumed him. The transformation was remarkable. Shane was so thrilled that he told me I should help others in the same way I had helped him. So, along with my son, James, who is a psychotherapist, I developed a course called "The Anxiety Algorithm," and we offered it to the people in our church. At the end of the first course, we followed up with the people who had attended, and 94 percent of them said their anxiety had improved. Numbers (when evaluated correctly) don't lie, and we knew that God had given us something special with this program.

The Philippians approach I presented to Shane and so many others isn't magic pixie dust. It's not a quick fix, and it won't get you back to feeling 100 percent all of the time. Past hurts and struggles take time to process, and life can be challenging. But this approach is special because it works, and it comes straight from Scripture.

Why do we call it the "Anxiety Algorithm"? An *algorithm* is "a step-by-step procedure for solving a problem or accomplishing some end."[1] Put simply, an algorithm is a plan. It's a solution to a problem. But, more than that, an algorithm can create a lot of good. It can make something beautiful out of something that is very broken. By learning to walk through the elements presented in Philippians 4 in the New Testament and other Scripture passages, you can quiet your anxiety and replace it with peace.

We will explore the Anxiety Algorithm plan in depth in coming chapters. But, first, it will be helpful to look at what wellness is and to learn some foundational practices and principles for reducing our anxiety and stress. In part 1, we will explore what it means to adopt a new way of thinking and living. In part 2, we will dive into the algorithm itself and how to personalize it to see the most effective results. In part 3, we will discuss how relationships impact our emotions, our anxiety, and how we think about ourselves. And, in part 4, we will look at ways in which, even with the inevitable difficulties and stresses that life brings us, we can live full lives that are characterized by joy and peace.

We offer *The Anxiety Algorithm* to all who are struggling with and suffering from anxiety, fear, and stress so they may increasingly move toward and experience the peace they have been seeking.

---

1. Merriam-Webster.com Dictionary, s.v. "algorithm," accessed October 7, 2024, https://www.merriam-webster.com/dictionary/algorithm.

1

BREAKTHROUGH MOMENT

I (James) will always remember the breakthrough moment a mother of three young children experienced during one of the Anxiety Algorithm classes my dad and I held at our church. We were explaining that this method must be practiced because, as with working out to lose weight and improve muscle tone, you can't expect drastic results immediately. As soon as we said this, the mother let out a fairly loud, "Really!" She explained that she had felt incredible guilt for continuing to struggle with anxiety even after asking God for help. In her mind, it was her lack of faith that was the problem, which had led to feelings of tremendous guilt and shame. This was someone who had walked with God for years, someone whom my father and I really respected for her Christian walk. She illustrates the many, many Christians who are struggling with an unspoken sense of guilt and shame because they cannot seem to shake the anxiety monster, despite their begging God to help them.

A PART OF LIFE

There is a dangerous mentality in the church today that assumes that if you're a strong Christian, you shouldn't be anxious. But that teaching is not found in the Bible!

Philippians 4:6 begins, *"Do not be anxious about anything,"* and we have a tendency to grab the first part of this verse and construct our mental health approach around it, thinking anxiety is a sin. But if you take a look at the context of the verse, you'll see that Paul himself admitted to having anxiety! Earlier in the book, he had been talking about Epaphroditus, who was his travel companion and who had almost died. We learn that the Philippian church had sent Epaphroditus to help Paul, and that everyone in that church was now concerned over the health of their brother in the Lord. Epaphroditus was distressed that his friends were so worried about him. So, when Epaphroditus recovered, Paul decided to send him back to Philippi. This would reassure the Philippians that Epaphroditus was well again, and it would relieve Paul's (and Epaphroditus's) anxiety over their deep concern. Paul wrote in Philippians 2:28, *"Therefore I am all the more eager to send him, so that when you see him again you may be glad and **I may have less anxiety**."* Some of Paul's anxiety may also have been due to the fact that Epaphroditus had taken risks doing the work of Christ. (See verse 30).

Paul didn't say that he was sending Epaphroditus so that he would have *no* anxiety. He said he was doing it to have *less* anxiety.

Putting this together, there is a clear message: anxiety is a part of life. It's something that we will experience from time to time. Having anxious thoughts or concerns is not a sin—it's to be expected. A cancer diagnosis is going to cause a certain amount of anxiety. A broken relationship, a wayward child, a major financial mistake—these things and more will cause anxiety.

Experiencing anxiety is not the problem. *But living in anxiety—dwelling in anxiety—is.*

This wasn't the first time in Paul's life that he had to navigate anxiety-inducing hardship. In Acts, we're told that handkerchiefs from Paul were sent around from community to community, and people were healed from their illnesses *just by touching these handkerchiefs*. Clearly, the hand of God was upon him, yet Paul also wrote this in 2 Corinthians 12:7–9: *"In order to keep me from becoming conceited, I was given a thorn in my flesh, a messenger of Satan, to torment me. Three times I pleaded with the Lord to take it away from me. But he said to me, 'My grace is sufficient for you, for my power is made perfect in weakness.'"*

Paul, the guy who was able to heal people via handkerchiefs, was unable to handle this *"thorn"* that gave him trouble. From what we know, Paul was never healed of the thorn. It was always there, a constant battle.

It's easy to come away from church with a misconception that if you do X, Y, and Z, all your problems will go away, but Paul shows us that's not how it works. There is not always a fix or solution to life's hardest things. But what we do have access to—and what Paul exhibited in all of his writings, despite dealing with the thorn in his side—is peace.

Jesus said in John 14:27, *"Peace I leave with you; my peace I give you. I do not give to you as the world gives. Do not let your hearts be troubled and do not be afraid."* And Joshua 1:9 reads, *"Have I not commanded you? Be strong and courageous. Do not be afraid; do not be discouraged, for the* Lord *your God will be with you wherever you go."*

You may be familiar with the saying "Practice makes progress, but Jesus makes perfect." Again, this book isn't going to solve all of your anxiety problems—that won't happen this side of heaven or until Jesus comes back. But it is possible to move toward wellness. It's possible to move toward peace. It's possible to have less anxiety and to learn how to live at your best even with a thorn in your side.

The only person you should be comparing yourself to is yesterday's you. If each day or week or month you get better than the one before, then that's progress. That's a life that's moving toward wellness.

WHAT ABOUT STRESS?

Stress has many effects, but let us agree it is uncomfortable. It gets us itchy, gets us wanting to change something in our lives. Stress paired with anxiety can be devastating, but it's important to understand that not all stress is bad.

There is a good kind of stress that will shape us. It will push us to make a change or adjust our approach for the better. It will pressure us to exceed expectations or to work hard on something. A great example of healthy stress is expressed in James 1:2–4: *"Consider it pure joy, my brothers and sisters, whenever you face trials of many kinds, because you know that the testing of your faith produces perseverance. Let perseverance finish its work so that you may be mature and complete, not lacking anything."*

All of us want to make progress in our Christian walks so that we don't lack anything that God desires for us. In fact, my dad and I tell our children (and grandchildren, in Ronnie's case) that we want them to be all that God has in mind for them to be. This is our definition of wellness, which we talk about more in the next chapter: becoming who you were created to be, a person who loves God and loves others and therefore loves themselves. Stress can help accomplish this. It can put us through the fire in a way that shapes us and changes us and moves us toward action and refinement. Our situation might be difficult, but we can find joy in our hope of how God is going to use it for His glory in our lives.

So, when does stress become unhealthy? When does a proper priority in life become a stressor? It's when what is most important in our lives is out of alignment. It is when we attach our ultimate hopes and security to anything other than Jesus, no matter how urgent or significant it might seem. It's easy to think that we know what our needs are, but Jesus very clearly spelled out for us our primary need. We may chase after different things, but He said, *"Seek first the kingdom of God and his righteousness, and all these things will be added to you"* (Matthew 6:33 ESV). This is a significant topic that we will talk about in more detail later in this book. Whenever we don't make God our first priority, we are welcoming stress into our lives. We can begin to drift, and our whole system of healthy priorities can get out of whack. But when we make God our first priority, we do not have to live in constant stress despite all of our other priorities and responsibilities.

God knows what we truly need, and when we seek Him first, we open ourselves up to receive from Him. When I (Ronnie) moved my family a few years ago, we decided to downsize. We hired three guys to help, and it took them six hours just to move the stuff from the attic! I had so much up there that I thought I needed but hadn't touched in years. What I had considered so necessary, so important, ended up costing me time and money to get rid of. By the time the move was completed, I had told the movers to throw it all away—to not tell me what the items were or what they had found—to just get rid of it. They loaded up a trailer with all that junk, and I haven't missed any of it since!

A similar scenario can be true of our spiritual, mental, and emotional health. We often think like the world around us: *If I can just have more money/if I can just have that person's job/if I can just have that person's looks, I'll be content.* But living like this just fills up our "attic" because we're always moving to the next thing, the next high, to fill the very real need we have for wellness in God.

What does that wellness look like? How can we clear away the stuff we have collected in our hearts and minds so we can move forward spiritually, mentally, and emotionally, living without continual anxiety or excess stress? We will explore this topic in chapter 2.

2

WHAT IS WELLNESS?

About 20 percent of the general population in the United States deals with clinical anxiety[2]—and that doesn't take into account the people who struggle with it but don't realize it. It's been reported that "an estimated 31.1 percent of U.S. adults experience any anxiety disorder at some time in their lives."[3]

With such a high percentage of people experiencing anxiety, even if you don't personally experience anxious thoughts or episodes, chances are you know a friend or a family member who does.

Living with anxiety—whether diagnosed or not—has become an almost normal, American thing. We hear people talk about their anxiety over leaving the house, making phone calls, attending uncomfortable business meetings, and making difficult decisions. And, as we saw earlier from Shane's experience, even the things in life that we are gifted in and equipped for—the good things, the things that are important to us—can become areas of apprehension for us.

---

2. "Anxiety Disorders," National Alliance on Mental Illness, https://www.nami.org/about-mental-illness/mental-health-conditions/anxiety-disorders/.
3. "Any Anxiety Disorder," National Institute of Mental Health, https://www.nimh.nih.gov/health/statistics/any-anxiety-disorder#:~:text=An%20estimated%2031.1%25%20of%20U.S.,some%20time%20in%20their%20lives.

A job that you have performed for years can suddenly cause you to feel crippling anxiety.

A relationship that seemed shaky but functional can suddenly trigger significant stress.

A routine action that you have done over and over for years can somehow feel mentally insurmountable to perform.

Entire books, courses, and careers have been given to analyzing and discussing anxiety, but we want to begin our discussion by approaching anxiety from a different angle—the healed and whole side of things.

Whether you're someone who has struggled with depression and anxiety or who knows someone who does, we want you to think about this crucial question: *What does it mean to be well?* What does wellness look like; what does it feel like?

Take a minute to think about that. Envision a well person, if you will. Imagine how they go about life, what their thoughts are like, and how they treat themselves. What do you see?

LOVING GOD, OTHERS, AND YOURSELF

In trying to tackle this very question of what it means to be well, I (Ronnie) began researching and reviewing scientific literature on the topic, and then I moved to theological literature. Eventually, I began talking to anyone and everyone who would engage with me about this subject. I asked questions and absorbed all the information and perspectives I could. I simply had to know what people thought about wellness—what it looks like and how it operates. I considered every viewpoint, every approach, every outlook, and I finally came up with what I consider the definition of wellness—and I found it in the Bible. I hadn't planned on finding it there. I had thought for sure I would find it in a medical journal somewhere, but the best glimpse of wellness that I could find came from Jesus Himself.

In Mark 12, a teacher of the law came to talk to Jesus. He had noticed that Jesus gave good answers to tough questions, and so he asked Him, in effect, "Tell me what the greatest commandment is." And so Jesus answered him by saying, "Hear, O Israel: The Lord our God, the Lord is one. Love the Lord your God with all your heart and with all your soul and with all your mind and with all your strength" (verses 29–30). It was a quote from Deuteronomy 6, a life truth that had gone back to Moses's time. It was as if Jesus was showing the teacher that His answer was no different from what the people of God had known to be true all along—that the best thing we can do is to love God with everything we have. Then, in verse 31, Jesus added that we should love our neighbors as we love ourselves. (See also Leviticus 19:18.)

I am convinced that this is wellness: to love God, to love others, and to love yourself. It's no simpler or more complex than that. How you love your neighbor is a pretty good indicator of how you love God. In fact, Jesus's final message to His disciples was similar to His statement about loving our neighbor. He told them to *"love each other as I have loved you"* (John 15:12). He could have reiterated any of the messages that He had given them over the years of His ministry: He could have told them to build the church, to feed the poor, to walk in humility, to care for orphans, or to keep their gaze on the kingdom. Instead, He told them to love everyone around them in the way that they had already experienced His love.

What does this mean? *Jesus understood that a person's wellness and right-mindedness hinges on how they love and receive love.* So, when we ask ourselves, "How is my wellness?" what we really should be doing is considering how we relate to and care for one another and how we relate to and care for God. These relationships—the relationship between you and others, and between you and God—make up the cornerstone of wellness. The way you give love to and receive love from God absolutely impacts the way you love others, which impacts the way you respond to and see the world around you.

"But, Ronnie," you may ask, "can it really be this simple?"

Yes! God never intended for life to be a riddle that we have to figure out or a puzzle we have to decode. He wants us to walk in health and oneness with Him—and He doesn't want to make that concept hard to understand. But while the answer might be simple, the journey to a life of giving and receiving love can be arduous.

AN AWARENESS OF GOD'S PRESENCE

Ultimately, we can receive and accept God's love only by being in His presence; we can do this by reminding ourselves about His various qualities, praying, worshipping, and in other ways. The more time we spend in His presence, the more we are transformed, enabling us to show love to others. That's what the Anxiety Algorithm is all about: *helping you move into a deep awareness of God's presence in your life.* So much so that, over time, remaining with Him and His peace will become the norm and not the exception in your life.

If this is true, if an awareness of God's presence produces wellness, and if it's also true that so many of us are still unwell…then, that must mean developing an awareness of His presence is *hard to do.*

We (Ronnie and James) believe that the Anxiety Algorithm unlocks a path to wellness through a process that guides us to receive God's love and to practice being in His presence. As we mentioned at the beginning of this book, an algorithm is a "step-by-step procedure and plan for solving a problem or accomplishing some end." This algorithm is not going to simply infiltrate your life as you read the words on these pages. And it's not a test that you can cram for or a quiz that you can fake your way through. It requires a day-by-day commitment to a different way of living, a different way of thinking. It requires practice.

Our role in this book is to usher you into an awareness of the presence of almighty God—a place where wellness occurs. And when you are in His presence—once you can put down the distractions and the busyness and the noise and truly sit with Him—all the stress that the world throws at you will start to fade away. Mind you, it won't fade in significance. The struggles you are going through will still be struggles. The hard things will still be hard. The ugly things will still be ugly. *But they will lose their ability to cause anxiety in your life.*

Don't you want this? Don't you need this? Don't you desire to experience God in a way that realigns your priorities and reframes your fears and worries? Don't you want to experience life with God instead of life on your own, where He may be only an afterthought for you?

God never intended for us to have to make this type of decision. The perfect world that He made for us to live, create, and thrive in had to be put on hold when human beings decided to follow their own desires instead of Him. Of course, it was Satan—the enemy of God—who originally tempted humanity, drawing us away from God's perfect plan, but it's almost as if we forget that this enemy is still at work today. He's still trying to chip away at our relationship with God. And one of the ways he does this is by attacking our awareness of God's presence. According to John 10:10, he comes into our lives to steal, kill, and destroy—and his primary target is our fellowship with God. He did it in the beginning, and he's doing it now—and the sooner we take that reality seriously, the sooner we can move to a place of understanding what is at stake and progress to a place of wellness.

To do this, we're going to approach anxiety in a couple of different ways. First, we will look at the neurological side and mental health issues. We'll talk about brain chemistry and the neural pathways of anxiety. And we'll see how we can move from being intentional to being reflexive (something we think is very important!), which allows us to handle life better. Along the way, we will provide you with tools and insights and practices, including various "Wellness Exercises," to help you to apply what you are learning.

It may seem as if we are giving you a lot of definitions, a lot of information, before we explore the Anxiety Algorithm in more depth in part 2. But this is because we all first need to build a foundation for wellness. We have to put in the time learning how to remain in God's presence, just as we spent years learning how to operate outside of it.

WELLNESS EXERCISE: DEEP BREATHING

It may sound rudimentary, but deep breathing is an extremely effective tool for addressing stress and anxiety, moving us from a troubled state into a calm state. Everyone has their own rhythm, but if you're new to this method, try this approach:

1. Inhale for four beats.
2. Hold for four beats.
3. Exhale for five beats.

If you're using the exercise for insomnia, you might inhale for six beats, hold for eight, and exhale for ten.

The science behind this is that by regulating the carbon dioxide and oxygen in your bloodstream, you will calm down. (And, to be honest, this is very similar to the method often depicted on television programs of anxious people breathing into a paper bag!) An increased intake of carbon dioxide reduces oxygen in your bloodstream, which helps to calm you down. This is what I mean: with deep breathing, you breathe in oxygen-rich air and hold your breath, giving your body time to use all of the oxygen and create carbon dioxide, then breathe out slowly. You just need to make sure that the time it takes to inhale is shorter than the time it takes to exhale, with a pause in between.

With enough practice, deep breathing can help to shut down panic attacks before they get out of hand.

Another breathing method is the physiologic sigh. This method is a bit easier to teach to kids:

1. Take two breaths back-to-back, without exhaling.
2. Exhale.

Do this four times, and you're likely to feel a bit better!

3

THINKING ABOUT HOW WE THINK

We're focusing specifically on the areas of anxiety, stress, and worry, but the concepts we talk about will apply to everything in our lives: every hangup, habit, or personal struggle. Any state of unwellness that Satan has caused or that you have allowed in your life can be worked out for good. God makes beauty out of ashes. He takes broken things and rebuilds them. He's the great restorer, and He longs to restore your life in the here and now as He builds His kingdom.

Throughout the Bible, there are stories about how God took something bad and broken and worked it out for the good. One of my (Ronnie's) favorites is the story of Joseph. He endured being rejected by his family, sold into slavery in a foreign land, falsely accused of a crime, and imprisoned, and yet God raised him up to a position of leadership that never would have been possible for one of Jacob's sons in the normal course of life. When Joseph was later reunited with his brothers—the ones who had set all this into motion by selling him into slavery—Joseph wisely said, *"You intended to harm me, but God intended it for good to accomplish what is now being done, the saving of many lives"* (Genesis 50:20). Joseph stayed in God's presence, and God took his hardships and turned them around in a way that blessed not only Joseph but also his family and the entire world.

Think about that! A story like Joseph's is possible for your life, too. You can experience closeness with God and clarity of mind even when life isn't fair. Even when it's painful.

HOW DO YOU DEFINE A SUCCESSFUL LIFE?

One hindrance to emotional wellness is accepting a false criterion for success, which can lead to burnout. One of the most startling realizations that a strong, Jesus-loving person can have is to suddenly recognize that they aren't abiding in Christ. Sure, they love Jesus and are saying and doing all the right things. Their intentions are good—but then they find themselves burned out. They end up stepping down from their ministry position, or they take a break from their church community to realign themselves. And then they charge back in—only to go through the same pattern. Rinse and repeat.

We (James and Ronnie) believe this happens when we look to the wrong things to determine whether we are "doing things right" in our lives. We're taught to look for fruit (see Matthew 7:16–20), but we interpret this to mean that we should look to other people's lives for markers of success as a sign that God's hand is on them, and try to emulate them. So, we see a large and growing church or ministry, and we imagine that the people running things are doing it right. We see a successful business run by a Christian, and we assume the owner must have a great relationship with God. We see a charismatic personality who seems to know God and the Bible, and we think, "Wow, look at that fruit!"

In looking for fruit mainly as indicated by prosperity, we often fail to check the branch that's holding the fruit—and we almost certainly don't check to see where that branch is grafted to the vine. The way someone abides in Christ, the way they sit in His presence, is what feeds the branch. That's what nourishes it, but we neglect to look there. We only have eyes for superficial manifestations of success, assuming that's all we need to know.

But stressed branches can make fruit, too.

Research from the Barna Group indicated that over 40 percent of pastors surveyed had considered leaving full-time ministry during the previous year. "Over half of pastors who have considered quitting full-time ministry (56%) say 'the immense stress of the job' has factored into their thoughts on leaving."[4] Part of this could be because Satan is attacking and discouraging pastors. Yet, at the same time, there are a lot of stressed branches producing fruit. There are even a lot of well-intentioned, Jesus-loving pastors who aren't adequately nourished, who struggle to abide in Christ, and who consequently become burned out. Many people don't realize how much their pastors need their support, both spiritually and emotionally.

I think most Christians struggle with what I (Ronnie) call "Old Testament Christianity," and which I define as a focus on works and on earning God's favor. (A performance mindset also afflicts people of all types of backgrounds, religious or not.) We think God blesses us only if we do well and produce results. But, often, God's blessings aren't what we think they are. It's only when we remain in Him that we can see His hand at work, blessing us with His presence, His peace, and His power. When we abide in Him, we see His plan more clearly. We understand that we don't *earn* blessings—we *learn* blessings.

The fruit we should cultivate doesn't look like packed-out churches and multimillion-dollar ministries and altar calls that draw vast numbers of people, although God does sometimes move through those means. The fruit that we should produce looks like what is described in Galatians 5:22–23 (ESV): "*Love, joy, peace, patience, kindness, goodness, faithfulness, gentleness, self-control.*"

Think of how much better your life would be if you had those qualities in abundance! This is the promise of wellness, of abiding in

---

4. "Pastors Share Top Reasons They've Considered Quitting Ministry in the Past Year," Barna Group, April 27, 2022, https://www.barna.com/research/pastors-quitting-ministry/.

Christ and being in His presence. As we move toward wellness, these fruits will grow in ways that will be obvious to everyone around us. It sounds amazing, doesn't it? But there is a tension that you'll have to work through to get there, a tension called "shame."

HOW DO YOU THINK ABOUT YOURSELF?

How we think about ourselves and our emotions can be another block to emotional wellness, especially when it leads us to think our mindsets and behavior are ingrained and can't be changed. *Shame* is a word rarely talked about in the church. We talk about feeling guilty over things we have done or things we should do but haven't, yet we don't usually talk about the shame we carry with us as a result.

Shame is a predator. While we can feel guilty over something we have done, shame comes in and tells us that we *are* that bad thing. It moves us from "I didn't treat my kids with love this morning" to "I am a terrible mother." From "I messed up and lied to my colleague" to "I'm a deceiver and a liar—no one should ever trust me." So, shame comes when we internalize our bad behavior, when we begin to believe that we are the horrible things that we do. In our minds, we become bad or wrong, going beyond having behaved in a particular way to being convinced we have a permanent character flaw. Real (not imagined) guilt can be helpful and akin to the biblical concept of conviction because it helps us to do the right thing. Shame is always harmful and akin to the biblical concept of condemnation because it makes us feel that God disapproves of us and that we are undeserving of any forgiveness or hope.

The very first emotion expressed by humans in the Bible is shame. The first human beings, Adam and Eve, sinned by doing something God had warned them against doing, and then they felt shame for what they had done. They skipped right from feeling convicted for their behavior to feeling shame for who they had become. And shame has been chasing us humans ever since.

As we work through anxiety, fear, or any other issue, it's important not to shame our emotions. Emotions are God-given. Feelings like sadness and hurt aren't condemned in the Bible, and emotions like anger and determination and confidence all have their rightful places as good and meaningful emotions when expressed in the right way. There's no such thing as a bad or wrong emotion. It's what we do with it that can be bad or wrong.

Accepting our emotions is the first step to learning how to take control of them. So, for the sake of this process, in which you are learning to release your anxiety and fear, it's important to accept that you will feel all sorts of things on this journey to wellness. You'll have emotions that feel good and emotions that feel uncomfortable or even wrong, and all of that is okay. It's part of sifting through the things that are hard so that we can better learn how to remain in Christ and bear the kind of fruit that is truly life-changing and freeing. It's important to trust that if we do our part, God will do His.

Effectively managing your emotions in order to function well in life is a key aspect of *mental toughness*, which is considered a mark of accomplishment and resilience.[5] Someone who has mental toughness has learned how to deal effectively with challenges, stressors, and pressure. They're able to put such things into perspective and shrug them off, to keep their head down and continue on even when arrows are being aimed their way. When they feel deeply, they're able to see their emotion for what it is and to allow that emotion to help them rather than hurt them. In this way, the emotion informs them rather than controls them.

But when you overlap this image of mental toughness with our scriptural idea of wellness, you come away with a much broader image of a healthy individual. When you add loving others as Jesus did to this goal of being mentally and emotionally strong, you end up with a powerful, purposeful person who is deeply caring and aware of others—you end up with someone who reflects the peace and strength of Jesus.

---

5. Simon C. Middleton et al., "Discovering Mental Toughness: A Qualitative Study of Mental Toughness in Elite Athletes," SELF Research Centre, University of Western Sydney, Australia, 2004, http://www.sectiononewrestling.com/discovering_mental_toughness.pdf.

4

THE SCIENCE OF ANXIETY

We've seen what the Bible says about anxiety, but what about science?

There's a very thick book published by the American Psychiatric Association that is the predominant diagnostic manual of mental disorders used in the United States. It categorizes anxiety-related disorders into two main groups. There are anxiety disorders, which cover social anxiety disorder, generalized anxiety disorder, and so forth. And then there are trauma- and stress-related disorders, which cover post-traumatic stress disorder (PTSD), acute stress disorder, and more. In this trauma- and stress-related grouping, there is something called adjustment disorder.[6]

Adjustment disorder is very common within mental health diagnoses. About 20 percent of the adult population may experience anxiety at any given time.[7] Many of these occurrences come from

---

6. *American Psychiatric Association: Diagnostic and Statistical Manual of Mental Disorders, 5th ed.* (Arlington, VA: American Psychiatric Association, 2013), 189–233.
7. "Any Anxiety Disorder," National Institute of Mental Health, https://www.nimh.nih.gov/health/statistics/any-anxiety-disorder.

stress-related problems, such as the death of a loved one or the loss of a job. When multiple stressors like these pile up at one time, a person becomes overwhelmed. Life is just too much for them to handle. Consequently, they develop anxiety and possibly unhealthy coping mechanisms.

Many people with anxiety have adjustment disorder due to stressors in their life. They've been through or are going through difficulties, and they start to experience symptoms of an anxiety disorder (adjustment disorder with anxiety) or symptoms of depression (adjustment disorder with depression) or both (adjustment disorder with anxiety and depression).[8]

On the other hand, many people struggle with debilitating anxiety that is not caused by stressors in their life (but stressors can absolutely exacerbate the anxiety). This level of anxiety impacts their ability to function daily. These individuals are diagnosed with a specific anxiety disorder depending on what the anxiety is centered on. For example, social anxiety causes obsessive thinking about failing to act or look "normal" in social settings. Generalized anxiety causes excessive worry about all kinds of things. For example, it may cause people to focus on the what-ifs of life or to fear experiencing the worst possible outcomes they can imagine. These types of anxiety are related more to one's predispositions and biological and genetic tendencies.

THE CAUSES OF STRESS

The causes of the stress are usually very specific, and we've discussed some of them above, such as the death of a loved one and job loss. See if you relate to any of these others:

Concern that something is physically wrong. This sometimes shows up as illness anxiety disorder, formerly known as hypochondria.

Concern that something is physically wrong with a loved one.

Financial issues. Money, whether lack thereof or risky financial betting, can cause serious stress.

---
8. *Diagnostic and Statistical Manual of Mental Disorders*, 265–290.

Lack of sleep. This is known clinically as *insomnia.*

Too much caffeine. Caffeine is a drug, and too much of it can exacerbate panic and anxiety. Withdrawing from a heavy reliance on caffeine can also trigger anxiety.

Improper use of medications. This can happen when a person is misdiagnosed or overusing or underusing their medication, and it's why doctors and psychiatrists have to be exceptionally careful about prescribing medications to children with ADHD. People can reach a point where they don't know if the issue is the medication or the illness—and they may not always know if they have an illness or if they are just experiencing a bad case of anxiety.

Improper diet and lifestyle. Consuming a large amount of carbohydrates and processed foods can affect how we feel, and a lack of movement can also trigger stress.

Performance-based mindsets. As a pediatrician, I (Ronnie) could always tell when a child's relationship with their parents was performance-based. They wouldn't come out and say it, of course, but they expressed that, usually, when they got home from school, the first thing out of their parents' mouths wasn't, "How was your day?" or "What was something fun that you did today?" It was often something like, "How did you do on that test?" or "How many points did you score at basketball practice?" And no matter how well the child did, it wouldn't be good enough. This tells the child that to be loved, they have to perform up to the parents' standards, and this can cause anxiety and stress for that child then and down the road. This is similar to an adult work environment that is consumed with results rather than value. Performance-based environments always encourage perfection—an impossible, anxiety-inducing expectation.

Relationship issues. Trouble in our friendships or marriage, or other issues with family, can wreak havoc on our minds and emotions, causing anxiety.

Unpleasant weather. If you've ever felt drained due to excessive heat or experienced the winter doldrums, then you've probably experienced the type of anxiety that weather can produce.

World crises. Chaos, war, and famine occurring in the world can cause us to feel hopeless and helpless. This situation is relatively unique in the sense that we can't do anything directly to solve these issues. We can't stop the wars or provide food to all the starving people, and so world crises, if we are invested in them emotionally or relationally, can cause us anxiety.

Loss of control. Any time that life moves in a way that is beyond our control, anxiety tends to rear its ugly head. It is much like being worried about world events, when it seems like there is nothing that can be done to solve the problem or to get life back on track. Such a sense of helplessness triggers anxiety for some people.

Information overload. Believe it or not, when you're browsing the Internet regarding a topic and receive fourteen million results—all vying for your attention and doing their best to distract you or even lead you in another direction—that is a stressful experience and certainly can cause anxiety.

Social media. We may use social media as an escape, but it can actually cause more anxiety than it does peace. Excessive use of Instagram, TikTok, Facebook, X, and all of the other platforms like them put users at an increased risk of anxiety—this includes you! Much as your primary care physician will tell you that you'll start to feel better if you lose five or ten pounds, most people start to feel better about life when they cut back on their social media time.

Research indicates that problematic or excessive social media use is associated with the following:

- Low self-esteem and social anxiety
- Negative social comparison
- Poor body image
- Depression

- Perceived social isolation
- Impaired cognitive and executive function
- FOMO (fear of missing out)
- Having an anxious approach to relationships
- Sleep quantity and quality[9]

If you struggle with one or more of the stressors mentioned in this list, your social media use is potentially contributing to your overall level of stress and anxiety.

We'll talk more about this later, but three primary symptoms have to be present for an anxiety disorder to manifest. They are: (1) anxious thoughts and feelings, (2) physiological symptoms/physical symptoms of anxiety, and (3) avoidant behavior. The last one especially has been exacerbated by the COVID-19 pandemic, the effects of which are still being felt by many people.[10]

A FALSE SENSE OF CONNECTION

Before the pandemic, we were forced to interact with people, to some extent. Churches usually only offered an in-person option, and the same went for jobs. Most grocery stores required you to go inside to shop, and going to the movies was something that many people did. But COVID-19 changed all that. Now, we can do almost everything from the comfort of our homes or cars. We've made our lifestyles more efficient or convenient, but we've lost connection with others—not only physically but also emotionally. We went from being asked how we are doing at least once a day to being asked how

---

9. Aviv M. Weinstein, "Problematic Social Networking Site Use–Effects on Mental Health and the Brain, *Front Psychiatry*, January 19, 2023, posted by the National Library of Medicine, National Institutes of Health, https://pmc.ncbi.nlm.nih.gov/articles/PMC9893026/#:~:text=Comorbidity%20with%20other%20disorders,and%20risk%20for%20problematic%20drinking.
10. Mayo Clinic Staff, "Anxiety Disorders," Mayo Clinic, May 4, 2018, https://www.mayoclinic.org/diseases-conditions/anxiety/symptoms-causes/syc-20350961#:~:text=Common%20anxiety%20signs%20and%20symptoms,avoid%20things%20that%20trigger%20anxiety.

we are doing once a week. Connection with others fills an emotional need that each of us has inside us—and it's harder than ever to find.

But it's not just the pandemic's fault. The chemical reaction in our brains that occurs when we view electronic screens gives us a *false* sense of connection with others.[11] This is particularly dangerous because we can be texting all day long and think that we're experiencing connectedness, when, in reality, that emotional need within us is still running on empty. Screens and technology give us the impression of emotional or relational intimacy without their actual benefits.

Some years ago, a seventeen-year-old girl came into my (Ronnie's) office with her mother. She was having significant problems sleeping, and I asked her to describe to me what was happening. She said that she had trouble falling asleep and that she couldn't get anxious thoughts out of her head. I then asked her to explain her nighttime routine, and I discovered that every night, she checked her phone. And she didn't just check it once—she checked it throughout the night. From her perspective, she was using her phone to help her fall asleep, making sure that she hadn't missed a text or an Instagram post from friends. But from my perspective, the phone was the problem because it wasn't allowing her to be in a frame of mind where she could rest.

I suggested that every night at nine o'clock, she put her phone in the kitchen and leave it there. Immediately, she started breathing hard. Then she broke out into a sweat and started trembling. She was experiencing a full-blown panic attack right there in my office.

This young woman had an intense emotional connection to her device. So much so that the thought of separating from her device for ten hours had caused her to experience physical symptoms of distress.

It was clear that she had such a dependent, unhealthy relationship with what she thought constantly checking her phone did for

---

11. Valentina Fernandez, "Social Media, Dopamine, and Stress: Converging Pathways," *Dartmouth Undergraduate Journal of Science*, August 20, 2022, https://sites.dartmouth.edu/dujs/2022/08/20/social-media-dopamine-and-stress-converging-pathways/.

her that limiting her phone use cold turkey would likely do her more harm than good. So, I switched gears. Once she calmed down, I asked her why my suggestion was so distressing to her.

"Someone may need me," she said.

"At two o'clock a.m.?" I asked.

"Yes." She was emphatic.

That was ten years ago, right around the time that social media was really picking up speed and becoming the norm. Imagine how much stronger the emotional connection is today for many people.

A very simple definition of addiction is when you give up something that's good for you to do something that's bad for you. This girl was addicted to her phone. She gave up sleep to use a device that was not helping her live a balanced life. It's easy to point a finger at her, but many of us struggle with the same thing today.

A cell-phone addiction may seem like a minor problem, but what happens when that addiction goes on for years? A Frontiers in Human Neuroscience article reported that chronic stress promotes inflammation in the body.[12] Inflammation is associated with many problems, including heart disease, cancer, arthritis, and some mental health conditions. Stress may also alter our metabolism. The chemical in the body that releases energy and produces the substances we need to grow, move, and stay healthy changes under stress. Stressful events can cause the body to burn fewer calories at rest. It can cause changes in our moods and increase our irritability with those around us.

There is a steep price to pay for the choices we make daily that contribute to unhealthy stress. So, let's look next at three words that will be crucial as we progress on our journey to wellness: *focus, think,* and *practice.*

---

12. Yun-Zi Liu, Yun-Xia Wang, and Chun-Lei Jiang, "Inflammation: The Common Pathway of Stress-Related Diseases," *Frontiers in Human Neuroscience,* June 20, 2017, posted by the National Library of Medicine, National Institutes of Health, https://www.ncbi.nlm.nih.gov/pmc/articles/PMC5476783/.

◇ ◇ ◇

WELLNESS EXERCISE: PROGRESSIVE MUSCLE RELAXATION

Progressive muscle relaxation (PMR) is an exercise that helps many people with anxiety.[13] We all carry tension in our bodies, and for those of us with anxiety, this tension really builds up and can become debilitating without our even realizing it.

With this exercise, you will progressively go through each muscle group, tensing the related muscles and then intentionally releasing them. By doing this, you're relaxing your muscles and addressing the hidden tension that is there. It's a great tool to use if you're having trouble falling asleep or if you find yourself in a position where anxiety is strong. For even better results, you can begin and end this exercise with deep breathing.

---

13. Loren Toussaint et al., "Effectiveness of Progressive Muscle Relaxation, Deep Breathing, and Guided Imagery in Promoting Psychological and Physiological States of Relaxation," *Evidence-based Complementary and Alternative Medicine*, July 2, 2021, posted by the National Library of Medicine, National Institutes of Health, https://pmc.ncbi.nlm.nih.gov/articles/PMC8272667/#B5.

As with any new exercise program, and especially if you have health problems, consult your health care provider before incorporating PMR.

Begin by finding a quiet, peaceful, and comfortable place to do the exercise. I recommend closing your eyes and doing a few rounds of deep breathing. Pay attention to your body and try to identify if you are feeling any tension. This may take a moment as you go through the different parts of your body. Then do the following:

- Spread your fingers by stretching each hand as much as possible, straightening the fingers and almost trying to make them bend upward toward the top of your hand. Hold this stretch for three or four seconds and then let your hand relax. Do this at least two times for each hand.
- Clinch your fists tightly and with effort for several seconds and relax. Do this at least twice.
- Flex your forearms for several seconds and then relax and repeat.
- Go back to your breathing and do the deep breathing cycle twice.
- Hold your arms in an X across your chest and tighten your upper arm muscles for several seconds, then release and repeat.
- Contract the muscles in your shoulders for several seconds, then release and repeat.
- Contract your neck muscles for several seconds, then release and repeat.
- Contract your face and scalp for several seconds, then release and repeat.
- Go back to your breathing and do two to three cycles of deep breathing. This time, imagine the tension in your body leaving as you exhale each breath.

- Contract your chest and stomach, hold for several seconds, then relax and repeat.
- Contract your upper and lower back muscles for several seconds, then relax and repeat.
- Contract your backside for several seconds, then relax and repeat.
- Go back to your breathing and, again, do several cycles of deep breathing while also imagining the tension in your body leaving as you exhale.
- Contract your thighs and hamstrings in your upper leg, hold for several seconds, then relax and repeat.
- Contract your calf muscles, hold for several seconds, then relax and repeat.
- Contract the muscles in your feet, hold for several seconds, then relax and repeat.
- Finally, flex your toes and extend them for several seconds, then relax and repeat.
- Return to your breathing and do several cycles of deep breathing. If you still feel some tension, you may need to continue imagining the tension leaving your body. You might even need to repeat the exercise until you do not feel tense.
- Now, when you breathe in, imagine breathing in the breath of life and the peace of God. Do this several times. As you exhale, say to yourself, "His peace goes with me."

5

FOCUS, THINK, AND PRACTICE

Every day, we are asked to make numerous decisions. These decisions create many different forks in the road or options we can choose. The two main decisions are these: we can go the way of the kingdom of God, or we can go the way of the world—meaning we embrace thoughts, priorities, and actions that are contrary to what God tells us is best for us and our emotional health. Sometimes the way of the kingdom is the easier, more appealing way. But, many times, it's the way of the world that that calls to us, that draws us. This is why we (James and Ronnie) stress the importance of focus, thinking, and practice.

Focus allows us to see these forks in the road. It helps us to recognize such moments for what they are. On the surface, they may seem so insignificant, so inconsequential. But kingdom things are often quiet things. Focus helps us to see them.

Thinking allows us to discern which way to go. Every day, you're going to have to decide one way or the other: "Will I do things in the kingdom way for God? Or will I do them only in a way that seems easiest or best for me?"

Putting focus and thinking into *practice* ensures that this process becomes habitual and that choosing the way of the kingdom becomes second nature to us, that it becomes who we are.

LET GO OF SEEKING PERFECTION

All this may seem like a formula for success, but what you'll find is that it actually frees you to make mistakes as you grow into wellness. It frees you to let go of seeking perfection and to start at the beginning, learning how to navigate life with Christ as your guide.

Hebrews 10:14 reads, *"For by one sacrifice he has made perfect forever those who are **being made** holy."* We are in process. We are being refined, being set apart so that our kingdom-focused lives can attract others who want to be a part of the kingdom. Perfection is not our goal. Abiding more in Jesus is our goal.

There is an account in 2 Kings 6 of an incident in which the servant of Elisha the prophet goes outside in the morning and sees the chariots of the enemy all over the hills. He rushes back to Elisha and says, "Oh no, my lord! What shall we do?" (verse 15). His fear was preventing him from seeing how God was moving in this circumstance.

Elisha tells the servant not to be afraid, saying, *"Those who are with us are more than those who are with them"* (verse 16). Then the prophet prays that God will open the servant's eyes so that he can see the protection God has sent them. The servant goes back, and he sees the hills full of chariots of fire: God's spiritual army sent for His people.

Unfortunately, many people live a defeated Christian life filled with stress, worry, and sadness because they are never satisfied with anything but perfection. We can't earn God's goodness and grace, and we certainly can't be perfect. But we can put all we have into learning and growing. There is excellence in effort, and there is faithfulness in waiting and trusting while you keep checking the hillside for God's army—and we hope that's what you will find with *The Anxiety Algorithm*.

THE PLAN, MOVING FORWARD

Think back to the greatest mentor in your life—the person who really helped you move toward wellness and growth. I (James) think of a guy named Phillip who came to our church as an assistant youth minister when I was in the eleventh grade. Phillip was about ten years older than I. I didn't have many friends who attended our church, and he took me under his wing and was a constant source of encouragement to me. Many times, I went to him to confess something that was bothering me, and sometimes it was no small thing that I had done or was caught up in. Still, Phillip's response was always the same: he would sit and listen intently, and then he would say something along the lines of, "Well, you know I love you," followed by something like, "What's the plan, moving forward?"

Even though there was always part of me that wanted to hide my sin because of the shame I was feeling, that sense of shame was never stronger than how good it felt to talk to Phillip and get things straight in my heart and with God. You see, Phillip inspired me to be a godly man. He believed in me, pushed me, and was quick to model Jesus's forgiveness and grace. He was never as concerned about my performance as he was about our relationship.

Jesus wants to be that kind of mentor to you. He wants to take on your shame, your striving, your inadequacies. He longs to intercede for you, to help you. But the only way He can do that is if you commit to changing the way you think and live. It's time to work on your relationship with Him, to consider Him in all that you do. It's not going to be easy. It's not going to be quick. It will take determination and perseverance to move closer to God and welcome more of Him into your life, but we are reminded of this in James 1:2–4: *"Consider it pure joy, my brothers and sisters, whenever you face trials of many kinds, because you know that the testing of your faith produces perseverance. Let perseverance finish its work so that you may be mature and complete, not lacking anything."*

Are you ready to put in the work? To focus, think, and practice so that you'll get to where you want to go, perfect and complete, lacking in nothing?

Yes, there will be friction. Beloved family members may try to dissuade you from moving forward, certain desires from within you may threaten to pull you off course, friends may not understand what you are trying to do, and old habits will be hard to change, but these types of friction are part of the journey. They are part of the process of shedding your anxiety and getting to a place where the friction doesn't bother you anymore. Where the most important thing that matters is the presence of God.

As you continue this journey with us, we hope that you will fully engage all of the material. We hope that you will spend time in daily prayer and Scripture memorization—we've found that to be especially helpful in our lives. And we hope that you will welcome others in on your journey. Perhaps there's someone in your life who can walk this process with you, keep you accountable, be a sounding board. Or maybe there's someone you know who could also benefit from learning about the Anxiety Algorithm. Reach out to them. See if they'd like to join you on this journey. You never know what might happen.

THE KINGDOM OF GOD IN YOU

In Galatians 5, Paul talks about walking by the Spirit, not by the flesh (our human tendencies that are influenced by sin and apart from God). He talks about living in such a way that you abide in Christ. We know that Paul struggled at times with acting in ways contrary to what he wanted to do as a follower of Jesus. In Romans 7, Paul wrote about doing things that he didn't want to do. While he was bothered by it, he didn't let it pull him down. He knew that God wasn't at all surprised by his humanness. Paul knew that Jesus would rescue him, and that He would redeem his life and make it whole. Can you imagine having the same perspective? Doesn't that sound freeing?

Let's remember that practice makes progress, but Jesus makes perfect. Yet Jesus said that the kingdom of God is within you. (See Luke 17:21 KJV.) *You!* Despite your anxiety and fears and doubts. Despite all of your flaws and shortcomings. Despite your tendency to produce fruit that will impress rather than fruit that transforms.

The kingdom is within you, and we're here to help you find it. To help you learn how to let it change you, transform you, so that you live in such a way that the kingdom of God not only remains within you but also emanates from you. To help you live a life of less striving, less perfection-seeking—and less anxiety.

6

ANXIETY, FEAR, AND THE "TWO STEPS BACK" STRATEGY.

As mentioned earlier, it's important to acknowledge that the word *anxiety* can be used to describe a disorder or a group of disorders, but it also can refer to an emotion or a feeling. A feeling of anxiety can be characterized by physical changes in the body, tension, worrisome thoughts, and increased blood pressure—and this feeling can hit any of us at times, whether we have an anxiety disorder or not.

A main difference between anxious feelings and an anxiety disorder is the presence of intrusive thoughts. These are thoughts that pop up uninvited and, more importantly, persist. When intrusive thoughts stick with you and become part of your life, this points more toward a disorder than a temporary anxious feeling.

Other differentiators are nervous sweating, trembling, dizziness, or a rapid heartbeat—all symptoms that are commonly associated with anxiety disorders rather than anxious feelings alone.[14]

---

14. "Anxiety Disorders," National Institute of Mental Health, reviewed April 2024, https://www.nimh.nih.gov/health/topics/anxiety-disorders.

People with anxiety disorders may avoid certain situations out of worry or fear, and many anxious feelings are rooted in some sort of fear. The American Psychological Association explains that "anxiety is not the same as fear, but they are often used interchangeably."[15] Much of the body's response to fear also happens when we face anxiety. The flight, fight, or freeze response can occur whether we are in a state of fear *or* anxiety. But to better differentiate the two, "anxiety is considered a future-oriented, long-acting response broadly focused on a diffuse threat, whereas fear is an appropriate, present-oriented, and short-lived response to a clearly identifiable and specific threat."[16]

REAL VERSUS PERCEIVED THREATS

I (James) used to work a lot with people who experienced anxiety when taking a test. These people were bright, knew the material backward and forward, and had no reason to be nervous, but once they sat for a test, anxiety would set in. It would get so bad that they would enter fight-or-flight mode. Now, the test itself wasn't a threat to them—it couldn't harm them—but their minds were convinced that the test was a danger. In this process of panicking over the test, their minds "erased" all the facts and data and information that they had studied in preparation for the test and instead focused solely on the perceived threat in front of them: the test itself.

Panic does this. It perceives something that is typically harmless as a threat, and it does this in a way that is no different from an actual life-or-death situation. This reaction can be very confusing to those who experience it.

To help these test-takers with anxiety, I'd work with them in several ways. I would educate them about the fight-or-flight system and their physiological and mental reactions, teach them deep breathing techniques, and work with their teachers to ensure that the students could keep their deep breathing instructions with them while taking

---

15. "Anxiety," American Psychological Association, https://www.apa.org/topics/anxiety.
16. "Anxiety," American Psychological Association.

the test. At the bottom of their instructions sheet, I'd write, "Look for the threat" to remind them that if they didn't see a grizzly bear or if there wasn't a fire breaking out in the building or a tornado on its way, then *there was no threat*, and they could do their breathing, regain their calm, and take the test.

I use the grizzly bear example regularly with adults because it so clearly shows anxiety and panic versus real, true danger and fear. When someone responds with fear to a picture of a bear, that's panic. There is no actual threat to them, but their mind reacts with fear and anxiety regardless. But when there's a real-life grizzly bear chasing you, that is a true life-threatening moment in which the mechanisms of fear (trembling, rapid heartbeat, focus on the situation at hand, and so forth) become very useful!

When you study fight or flight, you realize how only God could design such a system. This response involuntarily takes over your mind and body in an effort to keep you safe from real danger. But when this response is triggered in situations that aren't dangerous, it can do more harm than good.

So, when the thing triggering us is a picture of a grizzly bear instead of a real-life grizzly, we know there is a problem. When we feel fear creep up in situations that are more uncomfortable than they are dangerous, we need to take a step or two back.

THE "TWO STEPS BACK" STRATEGY

"Two Steps Back" is an important strategy that we'll use frequently in this book, and it comes from a time when I (Ronnie) took my grandkids to a wildlife exhibit. The presenter was talking about snakes, and he had all of the kids gather around a box. He reached in the box with a hook and pulled out the largest living rattlesnake in Mississippi (at that time) and held it up. It was slithering and rattling, and all the mothers in the room came to the front and pulled their kids away. It's a rule of thumb that if you come across a snake in the wild, it's best to take two steps back. You're not supposed to turn around and run or sidestep. You're supposed to take two steps back while facing the snake. This is because two steps put enough distance between you and the snake so that, if it tries to strike you, it will miss. If you waste time by turning around before you run or step to the side, that gives the snake just enough time to bite.

Taking two steps back from clear physical danger needs to be (and many times is) a natural reflex. But it's not always a natural reflex when it comes to danger that the mind has concocted.

I (Ronnie) remember when my wife was in a frustrating situation. She had let the region of her brain that processes emotion take control of her thinking, and she was beside herself with worry and anxiety. In order to be able to see the situation clearly, she needed to disengage that part of the brain and move her thinking to the top part of the brain, the higher level that allows you to think and reason and come up with solutions to problems. She did this by taking two steps back. Instead of becoming aggressive or complaining, she mentally stepped away from the situation and tried to look at it from a distance. This allowed her to take action that was effective and not just based on her emotions.

This method was so beneficial to her situation that we have adopted this Two Steps Back approach to every facet of our lives. When things get frustrating, when emotion—whether it's fear, anger, jealousy, or anything else—takes over, we take two steps back by removing ourselves from the situation long enough that we can think about what we want to say and what we want to do before we actually say or do anything.

A husband and wife who took our Anxiety Algorithm class told us that when they applied the Two Steps Back approach to disagreements in their marriage, they would often end up laughing about the thing that previously had them so upset earlier in the day! They quickly forgot why they had been so mad to begin with and were able to see clear paths through their disagreements.

Engaging the thinking part of the brain is what we're after. We want to move away from using emotion to handle regular, nonthreatening situations and instead use reason and intention to see things clearly and to determine a way through. Using the deep breathing exercise can help to calm us, allowing us to choose the Two Steps Back approach to restore peace to our emotions.

The Two Steps Back approach works because it helps us to avoid what has been called "the Hump."

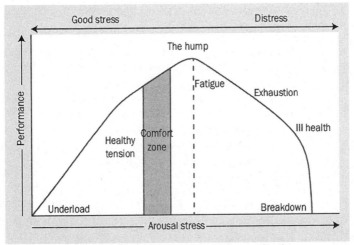

Human function curve. Source: Adapted from Nixon (1982)

The "Human Function Curve"[17] explains this concept. Good stress is a positive element in our lives. It's beneficial for us to use our minds and bodies to meet needs and to solve problems—problems even as basic as putting food on the table and finding shelter, or a place to live. This kind of stress motivates us to work, create, invent, and achieve. It motivates us to meet the needs of our bodies, minds,

---

17. Dr. Peter Nixon, a British cardiologist, introduced this concept. The chart on this page is adapted from Nixon's original graph by Toorban Mitra. See Mitra's article "Linkage of Job Ranks and Personality Traits with Augmented Stress: A Study on Indian Marine Engineers in the Context of the COVID-19 Pandemic," *International Maritime Health*, June 2023, 113, https://www.researchgate.net/publication/372193762_Linkage_of_job_ranks_and_personality_traits_with_augmented_stress_a_study_on_Indian_marine_engineers_in_the_context_of_the_COVID-19_pandemic. Used by permission.

and communities. If you have a healthy amount of good stress, you reach what is called the "Comfort Zone." This is the ideal state of being where you have just enough stress to keep you productive and to help you get off the couch and advance in life, but not so much that you become overwhelmed.

However, when added stressors enter the mix, that's when a person can be pushed outside of this zone. Stressors such as we discussed earlier—losing a job, receiving an unexpected medical diagnosis, experiencing grief or trauma, and so forth—can push a person out of the Comfort Zone, over the Hump, and into the area of "Fatigue." The real concern comes when someone remains over the Hump—when their life exists day in, day out in that area of fatigue.

The key is to prevent stress from ever reaching the Hump, and the two ways to do that are to:

1. Eliminate stressors from your life
2. Increase self-care

That's it. Do one of these, and you can prevent yourself from going (or staying) over the Hump. Sounds easy, right? The issue is that for an anxious person, this is a really difficult concept. Anxious people feel tense even in small things. Everything is a red-alert situation for them—everything is a stressor—and so, before they can sift out and remove the dangerous stressors in their lives, they have to learn how to see their situation clearly. They need to learn how to take Two Steps Back.

THE HUMP

Over thirty times in twenty chapters, the book of Luke mentions that Jesus retreated for silence, solitude, and prayer. He exercised self-care in a major, effective way! It was necessary to His ministry, to His relationship with the Father, and to His mental health. He was self-aware enough to know when He needed to take time to center Himself.

You can do this, too. When you see the stressors in your life build up, you can counteract them by increasing your self-care. For example, you can exercise six times a week instead of three. You can go to bed an hour early each night. You can eat more nutritious foods and spend more time with friends who build you up and less time in front of the TV. It's when we let life happen to us that we become distressed and fatigued, and we need a greater level of assistance—more than anything we can provide on our own.

Some people may even experience a major depressive episode with some level of psychosis when they reach this state of prolonged fatigue. These are people whom you may never expect to have a mental break, but, the next thing you know, they've checked into a behavioral health facility because they need expert care. They need a bigger team to help them figure out what got them there and how to get back over the Hump. They need professional help to take Two Steps Back.

It is important to note here that not everyone who experiences clinical depression or anxiety is symptomatic just because they are over the Hump. Some people are at higher risk for these syndromes and can experience episodes of anxiety or depression despite being very healthy and pursuing wellness. We are saying that staying over the Hump will eventually lead to burnout and likely bring about unwanted symptoms.

One of our goals is for this algorithm to help you recognize when you're on the side of health and when you're on the side of unhealth. We want you to not become anxious about being anxious and to learn how to live in balance in the space in front of the Hump. And, we hope you are able to walk yourself back to the Comfort Zone should you ever find yourself on the edge of the area of Fatigue.

This is especially important if you are a performance-based person. Performance-based people tend to live close to the Hump, right on the verge of having too many stressors in life with not enough self-care. Before they know it, they're not sleeping well, not feeling rested. They feel more sluggish than normal. The things that drove and excited them seem less appealing and more stressful than they did the previous month. When you can spot the symptoms, you can take Two Steps Back and rearrange your approach. Again, you can ask friends for support, spend more time exercising, take an afternoon off to recharge spiritually—whatever it takes to get back on the other side. But to spot the symptoms, you need to become well-versed in taking Two Steps Back.

SO HOW DO WE DO THIS?

Taking Two Steps Back incorporates the *focus*, *think*, and *practice* steps, but in a very targeted way.

First, take a moment to be by yourself with little or no distractions. *Focus* on the situation at hand. Try to visualize other people in the same situation as opposed to seeing yourself in it.

Then, you'll want to *think* about what to do. Continuing to visualize other people in the same circumstance, think about what would be the easiest way, the most beneficial way, through the conflict. What would you tell those people? How would you advise them? How do you think Jesus would handle this situation? What is a kingdom response? What does Scripture say?

Last (and this step doesn't need to happen right away; there is benefit in waiting for the right time or for the Lord to speak and reveal the best way through), you'll want to *practice* choosing the way of the kingdom in whatever situation you're facing.

You can see that the Two Steps Back approach is really about making room for God's Spirit to speak to you and to guide your actions and words.

WHAT ABOUT THERAPY?

As we focus, think, and practice using the Two Steps Back method, it's important to remember that the type of stress that gets you to run from a grizzly bear is good stress. Good stress is also the type that urges you to do your best when preparing and giving a presentation or to quickly rearrange your day so that you can rush to school to pick up your sick child. But the type of stress that anxiety creates is always negative. It always hurts; it doesn't help you grow or become a better follower of Jesus, even though your brain may tell you otherwise.

Some of the best therapies that we have for helping people who are anxious come under a category that's called cognitive behavioral therapy. This approach focuses on the intersection of *cognition*, representing the thinking side of us; *behavior*, representing our habits and tendencies; and *emotion*, representing our feelings or emotions. You can think of this as a triangle, with each aspect impacting the other.

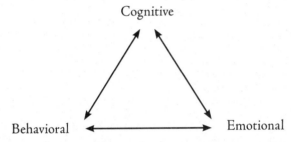

Each of these aspects affects the others. Behavior can affect your thoughts and emotions. Emotions can affect your behavior and thoughts, and your thoughts can affect your emotions and behavior. Because each impacts the others, it's not helpful to simply tell someone, "Hey, stop feeling so anxious!" because anxiety isn't just an emotional issue; it's a cognitive and behavioral issue as well.

In a therapy situation, changing the way someone is *feeling* is very difficult; it is much easier to help someone by assisting them to change their *mind*, their *thoughts*, and, eventually, their *behavior*, targeting the way they respond to things.

We'll touch on this more later in the book, and we will also provide you with the full algorithm to help you gain mastery over worrisome thoughts. We have seen incredible changes in people who have journeyed with us, and we believe that if you will fully engage with the algorithm, your anxiety and even your life overall will improve. But in addition to the algorithm, the Two Steps Back approach, and any other advice we're offering in this book, please know that it is in many cases good and right to journey through this process with the help of a licensed therapist. This is especially true if you are someone who deals with depression. Depression is such a chemical-brain issue that it's simply not fair to tell someone who struggles with it to change their mindset or to take Two Steps Back. Depression and moderate-to-severe anxiety issues require therapy and often even medication in addition to the tips and advice that we offer in this book. Therapy will even help if you deal with a milder form of anxiety or depression. So please know that if you struggle with diagnosed depression or anxiety, please continue on the path of wellness that your health care providers have advised for you. This book will help, but it should not be your only tool.

GIVE IT A TRY

Do you want God's peace or the world's form of peace? This is a serious question if you're someone who has a tendency toward anxiety or has an anxiety disorder. Do you want peace that is within and that lasts for eternity, or peace that comes and goes based on whatever life hands you on a given day? When you're struggling with anxiety, it can feel as though your brain is out to get you, but there is healing in Jesus. Taking Two Steps Back is a huge part of allowing God to work and move in your thoughts, fears, and worries. All you need to do is to give it a try. The next time you feel anxious, take two steps back. You may find that the God of peace—who is with you at this very moment—provides immediate relief. Or, you may find that this road is going to be a lot longer than you anticipated. That's okay, too. We often need to go through a process to find healing, and you can know that the God of peace is with you throughout your journey. (See, for example, Hebrews 13:20–21.) We are also here with you for the ride—and we have plenty more to share.

WELLNESS EXERCISE: SELF-CARE

Self-care is a hot topic these days—and for good reason: it is about trying to have balance across all areas of our lives.

SELF-CARE GRAPH

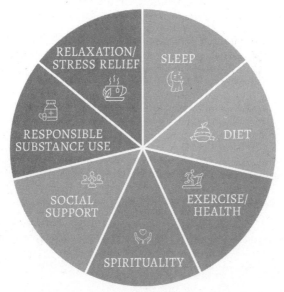

The sections of the graph will help you evaluate and work on your self-care. Every day, take one of these sections and be intentional about it. This is a good way to encourage self-reflection and self-awareness while working on finding a better balance of mind, body, soul, and strength.

You might approach the categories like this:

Sleep: How much sleep do I get? Does it feel like I am getting enough, or am I always tired? How would my life be different if I were to set consistent sleep hours?

Diet: Do the foods I eat nourish my body? Do I eat when I'm hungry, or do I eat when I'm stressed/anxious/sad/etc.? How often do I cook at home versus eating out? How different might my body feel if I focused on eating a more balanced diet?

Exercise/Health: How often do I move? How can I add more movement to my day? Am I too obsessed with or too avoidant of fitness? When I think of the hours in a day, does this category get too much or too little of my time?

Spirituality: How much time per day do I spend with God praying, reading, sitting in silence, etc.? How much time do I want to spend with Him? How can I make that happen?

Social Support: How often am I with friends and family in person? How might my life change if I spent more time with people who build me up and encourage me toward God and toward wellness?

Responsible Substance Use: How often do I smoke, drink alcohol, need caffeine to function, and/or use recreational drugs? Does it feel balanced or out of balance? Are my substance use practices healthy for me? Do I need these things to unwind, or am I capable of going without them? What might God be calling me to do in this area?

Relaxation/Stress Relief: What do I generally do to unwind? Does that habit truly help me to relax, or does it just temporarily shut out my worries/anxiety? How might my life be different if my relaxation time was planned out and focused on things that are truly relaxing and life-giving?[18]

If we are living in a balanced way when life is slow and quiet, then we have a better chance at staying balanced when life is chaotic, busy, or hard.

---

18. See Lisa D. Butler, et al., "Six Domains of Self-Care: Attending to the Whole Person," *Journal of Human Behavior in the Social Environment*, 29(1), 107–124, https://doi.org/10.1080/10911359.2018.1482483.

7

◇ ◇ ◇

HEALING BROKEN HUMANS

I (Ronnie) am one of those Christians who started going to church nine months before I was born. I've never known life without church and God, and from the time I was a child, I've been very active in my church community. But when I was about eight years old, I decided that I didn't want to go to church anymore. Every Sunday, I'd tell my parents that I wasn't going, but they would make me go anyway, saying that it didn't matter how I felt. Going to church was what we did.

My dad used to love to listen to gospel music, and, at that time, I'd even tell him to turn off his music, that I didn't want to hear it. It made me feel uncomfortable, uneasy. There was something about the music and church and the Bible that seemed at odds with my eight-year-old heart and mind.

I remember one Sunday morning when I asked my mother what was wrong with me. "Why don't I want to go to church anymore? Why does it bother me so much?" And my wise, wonderful mother looked at me and said, "I think you're finally understanding that there is something separating you from God, and that's called sin." She went on to explain that Jesus's death on the cross made it possible for me to get rid of that sin so that I could be in the family of God. Sin, the thing that was making me feel uncomfortable and unworthy of God's presence, could be erased, and I could find joy when I entered God's church—His family—reconciled to Him.

Right then and there, I prayed that God would forgive my sin and allow me to become part of His family. From that point, my relationship with church changed. I felt accepted and included. I felt that God was right there with me. He wasn't some Being hovering somewhere far off that I couldn't reach.

I wish I could say that my relationship with God has been strong ever since, but there have been hills and valleys within it. For the most part, prayer and Bible reading have been a steady part of my life, but when I started a pediatric practice, everything blew apart. I was stretched very thin, and things that had been routine in my life for years were being left behind. Praying and reading Scripture became practices that I hoped to be able to do again one day but I couldn't make time for while I was juggling so many other important things. I was too busy, too frantic, too tired. My life stressors went over the Hump, and my spiritual life began to drift.

I firmly believe that if you don't steadily read the Bible, your relationship with God will suffer, and I felt that effect immensely. Suddenly, things were harder for me, and life was more of a struggle. Not because the things that I faced were worse than before, but because I lacked peace, joy, and hope. I was trying to do it all on my own instead of relying on the presence of God in my life.

I was convicted about this, but I didn't know how to correct my course. I was getting up at all hours of the night, going into the hospital, running on fumes while trying to build a successful practice, and I remember crying out to God in my distress. I wanted more of Him in my life but could not see a way to make that happen.

I felt God say to me, *What is something you do every day?*

"Eat," I thought. "I eat every day."

And God said, *If you can take care of your body by eating food, then you can take care of your spirit by eating spiritual food.*

"Okay, I can do that," I decided. So, each day, I committed to refrain from food until I had read some Scripture.

I'd like to say that God parted the waters and made it possible for me to fit Scripture into my schedule, but that's not what happened. The process was messy and imperfect, but I made it happen. There were days when I read my Bible while in the bathroom! Days when I was grabbing passages as I could between patients. Days when I ended up not eating for hours and hours because life was so frantic that I couldn't find a moment to be in the Word.

But here is what happened: the passages that I was able to sneak in here and there nourished me. My anxiety and depression lifted. My peace came back. I felt centered again. The circumstances of my life had not changed—I was still operating on little sleep and a lot of fumes—but because my spirit was nourished, my mindset shifted.

Moving toward wellness is about putting good habits into practice. It's about choosing things that nourish over less important things that are vying for our attention. But this is hard to do when our priorities are out of balance.

A Barna Group survey conducted between December 2022 and January 2023 gathered the thoughts of American teens and adults regarding what they look for in their spiritual beliefs.[19] The survey is fascinating, and we highly encourage you to look it up, but there were a few takeaways that we want to share. We believe these show the perspective of most people in our culture.

The participants were asked to rank in order of importance the things that they wanted out of spirituality. Their options were "inner peace," "hope," "healing," "forgiveness," "truth," "purpose," "guidance," "growth," "meaning," and "salvation."

---

19. "Peace, Hope, Healing—What Spirituality Means to Americans Today," Barna Group, April 5, 2023, https://www.barna.com/research/spirituality-means/#.

Of those ten options, hope and inner peace ranked highest across the board, whether a person was a Christian, someone of another faith, or an atheist. Most people, including people of other faiths and people with no faith, want peace and hope in their lives more than anything else. They crave it; they seek it. Peace and hope are universal needs and desires, and yet we struggle to prioritize the things that can bring us true peace and hope. What's worse, our anxiety and depression actively steal away our peace and hope.

This isn't a new problem. It started all the way back in the garden of Eden.

IN THE BEGINNING

The story of the garden of Eden is significant for understanding the root causes and issues of anxiety so we can address it. In Genesis 2:18, God looked at Adam and knew that things would be better if Adam had a helper and suitable companion. That verse marks the first time God said something was *not* good—everything else up to this point He had declared good. (See Genesis 1.)

Our English translation does not do justice to the original Hebrew word translated as *"helper"* in this verse. The original intention behind the word was a military concept, and a better translation would be "powerful advocate." In creating Eve, God intended her to be a partner who would be willing to go into battle, who would be willing to fight by Adam's side.

In Hebrew, the word used for *"suitable"* in the text hints at someone who is an *equal-opposite*. God created Eve to be different from Adam—unique, and just as valued and just as important in her own way.

An equal-opposite. A powerful advocate. That was the role of Eve, and, in a sense, it is the role of all those who are in Christian community.

Most of us who are married would acknowledge that we are not like our spouse, and our spouse is not like us. I know that if I

(Ronnie) were married to someone exactly like me, we'd be living in a hut somewhere! My wife keeps me organized and able to do what I believe God has called me to do. She is absolutely a powerful advocate, an equal-opposite.

Scripture tells us that Adam and Eve—in their equal-opposite relationship—walked with God in the cool of the day. (See Genesis 3:8–10.) They physically walked with their Creator, but they also had a relationship with Him. They were in His presence in the garden and were very close to Him. The Bible also tells us that they were naked and felt no shame. (See Genesis 2:25.) This is important because while they were physically naked without shame, it also hints at the fact that they were transparent before God. They were open and honest in their relationship with Him and held nothing back. God saw them as they were, no shame involved.

As we pointed out earlier, shame is at the root of most relational and mental health issues, and it brings anxiety. Yet, in the garden, Adam and Eve didn't struggle with either of those things. They had no shame or anxiety, and they had an intimate relationship with God.

Until Satan came along.

A LOST SENSE OF CONTROL

Satan found Eve in the garden and began to talk to her. He started picking at her relationship with God, causing her to doubt what God had told her. God had said she would die if she ate the fruit of the Tree of Knowledge of Good and Evil (see Genesis 2:17), but Satan said that fruit would open Eve's eyes and give her godlike knowledge (see Genesis 3:4–5)—and who doesn't want to be like God?

Authority and power were given by God to human beings in creation, and exercising that authority is a natural human desire, but Satan appealed to this desire in an unhealthy way in order to undermine Eve. He uses the same tactic today to get to you and me.

A lot of the anxiety we experience comes from a sense of having lost control. Despite being loved and cherished by a God who is in control of all things, we want to take the wheel and call the shots. When that doesn't work, and when our false sense of control is gone or dwindles, we start to spiral downward, and the what-ifs of life, the uncertainties, get to us.

This is exactly what Satan wants. If he can get us to believe that God really isn't in control, that the universe is just as much under the rule of chaos and evil as it is under the rule of God, then we start to lose our trust in God and step away from His presence. We begin to look to other things to help us feel in control again, and since other things cannot help us the way God can help, we descend into anxiety, fear, and depression.

Eve experienced this. She bought the lie that things would be better if she were calling the shots, and she ate the fruit. Don't kid yourself, though. She didn't act alone. Adam watched this happen. He could have stepped up and stopped it, but he did nothing. Eve gave some fruit to Adam, who ate it, and their eyes were indeed opened—but in a negative way. (See Genesis 3:6–7.)

If you're a parent, you've most certainly, at one point or another, told your kids not to go into the cookie jar. When they disobey, it's not always pretty. You're upset—hurt, frustrated, and disappointed. At the time, it may be difficult for you to see past these emotions, and you may express them, and perhaps you send your child to their room for a time-out. But God's response to Adam and Eve going into the cookie jar was completely different: He went looking for them with the intent of lovingly drawing them back into His presence. He called to Adam and Eve, "*Where are you?*" (Genesis 3:9).

Of course, He was aware of where they were hiding, but still He patiently called and waited, even though He knew that what they had done had changed them in a way that would bring darkness and suffering into the world and take millennia to make right. Can you feel His compassion?

God called to Adam and Eve in order to help them understand where they were in a spiritual sense. After a life spent in the presence of God, for the first time, Adam and Eve were alone. They were no longer walking and talking with their Creator—they felt the need to hide from Him.

The second thing God did was to ask if they had eaten the fruit. Again, God knew what they had done, but He also understood the importance of allowing them to come forward with the truth.

Adam and Eve's initial response to their sin was to cover themselves, because they suddenly felt shame. Their shame was based on comparison. They realized that they were different from one another, and *different* took on a whole new meaning after the fall. Different was no longer seen as beautiful; it was no longer celebrated. Instead, different meant unequal.

Author and pastor Timothy Keller ministered in Manhattan for many years, and he was famous for saying that many people in New York are trying to use "fig leaves" all the time. They're trying to cover up the differences that make them feel less than worthy as people.[20] Doesn't that just hit home?

Adam and Eve's differences pulled them apart and caused them feelings of shame and comparison. Furthermore, they began to look at their relationship with God through the lens of performance, not fellowship. There was no longer the intimate relationship of walking with God in the cool of the day. They thought that since they hadn't performed the way God wanted them to, He would stop loving them. The security and safety in God's love they had felt before the fall had crumbled as they doubted His goodness, doubted His love.

Today, many of us struggle with the same things. We think that God expects certain things of us, and if we don't do those things, He will remove His hand from our lives or take our names out of His Book of Life. We think that He no longer wants to walk with us in the cool of the day.

---

20. Timothy Keller, "Paradise Lost," sermon, Gospel in Life website, June 23, 2023, 34:59, https://podcast.gospelinlife.com/e/paradise-lost/.

The Bible is clear that there's nothing you can do to make God love you more, and there's nothing you can do to make God love you less. The beautiful relationship He had with Adam and Eve before the fall? He wants the same with you. This is what grace is for, and God offers it to us completely and totally through Jesus Christ. But Adam and Eve could no longer see God's grace clearly, and they began to grasp for control. Sound familiar?

GOD IS LOOKING FOR US

God made us in His image, but we tend to skip over that reality. (See Genesis 1:26–27.) He put a part of Himself into us so that we could have a living soul: *"And the LORD God formed man of the dust of the ground, and breathed into his nostrils the breath of life; and man became a living soul"* (Genesis 2:7 KJV). We are walking, talking representations of the God of the universe, and Satan can't stand that idea. Not only that, but he'll do everything he can to destroy our representation of God and His nature; and, if the world around us is any indication, he's doing a decent job of it. God is in control, but Satan has wreaked havoc in hearts and minds, bringing about unprecedented levels of shame and fear, starting with Adam and Eve and continuing through the centuries and millennia to us.

But the reason we were created in God's image is for relationship with the Divine One. Sin and the fall drastically altered that relationship, but God's heart for it has remained the same.

Regardless of God's love for His creation and His desire to be in relationship with human beings, people keep piling on the shame and hiding from Him. We've come to a place in the church where we can't even say the word *sin* without people getting upset. Talking about sin makes people feel bad about themselves. It brings shame because we know we have issues, we know we have problems, but we don't want to face them. It's too painful.

In my (Ronnie's) years as a doctor, I saw patient after patient who came to me with a serious concern, only to say that they had known about it for a while but hadn't done anything about it. In some of these cases, we were able to get them fixed up, and the only unfortunate part of it was the time they had wasted suffering from their ailment while getting up the courage to come to see me. In other cases, we weren't able to help as much as we would have if they had come sooner!

Similarly, so many of us live our lives hoping that our sin will go away on its own. Hoping that our shame can be kept safe and unexposed. Meanwhile, God is in the garden, looking for us. "Where did you go?" He calls.

God went looking for Adam and Eve so that He could begin to restore their relationship with Him, and He looks for us for the same reason.

We must realize that nothing we read about in the Bible about the fall of humanity was a surprise to God. From the beginning, God had a plan to redeem us to Himself. He knew we would fall away and that He would enact His plan to restore us. His reasoning for this is made clear in Ephesian 3:10–12:

> *His intent was that now, through the church, the manifold wisdom of God should be made known to the rulers and authorities in the heavenly realms, according to his eternal purpose that he accomplished in Christ Jesus our Lord. In him and through faith in him we may approach God with **freedom** and **confidence**.*

So, in a sense, we're on stage. As we participate in God's plan, we show the heavenly realm what God is all about. God is making things right, giving human beings a way to enter back into His presence. Yet, just like Adam and Eve, we run and hide from Him. We could walk with God in the cool of the day. We could have the freedom and confidence that He offers—after all, He lives in us! He is always with us. Yet we choose separation. We choose to do things our own way. We choose to try to control things "like God does," but that choice to do it on our own only leads to anxiety and fear.

The cost of God's reconciling us to Himself was the life of His Son. Once more, God knew this would be the case, even when He chose to create us. He knew how things would unfold, and yet He chose us anyway. He gave everything. He gave Himself.

It's time for us to daily choose Him.

In the anxiety, the fear, the shame, and whatever else Satan throws at you, you will stumble. You will make mistakes. But you must keep moving toward God, toward wellness. This isn't something that you'll master overnight. It takes time to get to a point of deep shame and deep anxiety, and it takes time to get out of those feelings and into wellness.

The only thing we're asking of you is that you practice moving toward Him.

8

MOVING TOWARD GOD AND WELLNESS

It can be hard to accept the idea that God kicked Adam and Eve out of the garden after their big mistake. Despite His love for them, and despite the fact that He is a God of second chances, He drew a clear line. (See Genesis 3:8–24.) He didn't kick them out to punish them, though—that's never His aim. He did it to enact His plan.

You see, the garden was perfect. It was literally heaven on earth. Adam and Eve were now sinful. So, imagine a perfect creation with sinful humans in the midst of it. The two do not go well together. The garden wasn't going to help Adam and Eve deal with their newfound sin any more than it helped them prevent the sin in the first place. God knew that they needed a fresh start. He moved them out of the garden so that He could begin His process of restoration. He knew that the only way for Him to reach them at the soul level was for them to be out in the world beyond the garden. You see, when life is going well, when things are working out and everything is in line (much like life in the garden), our sinful nature (which is what Adam and Eve both had at this point) makes us drift from God. We think that we've got things figured out and don't need Him. A life in the garden would have absolutely triggered this! It would not have pushed them toward God but away from Him.

God's plan was to allow Adam and Eve to live in a fallen world where there is hardship and pain and suffering and also a strong need for Him. He intended for them to grow in community, in togetherness, and He would be right there with them and their descendants, generation after generation, always working toward reconciliation.

The story of reconciliation climaxes when a tree of death became the tree of life: Jesus died on the cross for our sins and rose again, conquering both sin and death. Having done so, He gives life to all who will receive Him. John 1:12 says, *"Yet to all who did receive him, to those who believed in his name, he gave the right to become children of God."*

We need to pay especially close attention to this next verse because it directly applies to managing and overcoming our anxiety. Philippians 4:19 says, *"And my God will meet all your needs according to the riches of his glory in Christ Jesus."*

When we truly believe this, we can address our anxiety. When we fully believe that God will provide and that He knows what's best, then we finally begin to experience the peace that He brings. We stop trying to control what we will eat, where we will work, how our career is going, and what people think of us. We trust Him with the dangers and obstacles in our path, and the fear of those things does not consume us.

The parable of the prodigal son is one of Jesus's most well-known parables. In this story, a young son does everything against his father's will. He takes his inheritance, leaves his family, and does whatever he wants with his life, which leads to brokenness and despair, anxiety and depression. But when the son comes crawling back home, the father welcomes him wholeheartedly and treats him as if nothing had happened. And that's what God does for us.

A life apart from God's presence—a life on our terms—does not satisfy. It leads to consequences that bring anxiety and depression.

But a life lived in the presence of God provides the peace of mind to weather the difficulties of life with hope and joy.

In my (Ronnie's) pediatrician practice, we administered countless vaccines for children, and I always saw the same pattern. A new baby didn't think anything of getting a shot, and so the first few rounds of vaccinations were always fairly simple for the child and their parents. But by the time the child reached fifteen or eighteen months, they knew what was coming. As soon as they saw the nurse enter the exam room, they started screaming and crying, doing everything they could to get out of the vaccination. The child saw us doctors and nurses as the problem. From their perspective, we hurt them, and they wanted nothing to do with us.

The hardest of all were the preschool shots. The children were old enough to be aware of what was going to happen. They also had a close relationship with their parents. They knew how much they loved their parents and how much their parents loved them. They trusted them. So, why in the world would someone with whom they were in that kind of relationship allow so much pain in their life? Why would their loving parent hold them down to let someone poke them with a needle (sometimes up to three times!)? Children of that age do not understand the science behind vaccinations. They do not understand that their parents are "causing it to work together for good." (See Romans 8:28.) Later, as the children matured, it all made sense. But not at that moment. All they could do was trust their parent, and that was hard.

I remember a mother who had to hold her child's leg so that we could administer a vaccine. Tears rolled down her face, but she knew the importance of that vaccination. She knew what was best for her child even though it was difficult for her.

I saw Jesus in her that day. I saw a reflection of our loving Lord and Savior, who says, "I'm taking this hard, painful thing in your life, and I'm going to make something beautiful out of it. I don't like these hard things any more than you do, but stick with Me, and I will make it right. I'm building you up for My kingdom—I've got an important assignment for you." When we start to view God through His love, everything shifts.

But here's the catch within this medical analogy, in which the difficulties we go through are like vaccines that strengthen our bodies against the effects of disease: even vaccines are not 100 percent guaranteed. No vaccine can provide full immunity. Sometimes, a vaccinated person contracts the very disease that they were supposed to be protected against. But to catch something, you have to be exposed to it. This is why mass vaccinations are so important. The more people who are vaccinated, the less likely the chances of their catching something. This practice helps to protect those who are the most vulnerable. When all of us are vaccinated, then the likelihood of even the most vulnerable among us contracting a disease goes way down.

The same idea is true of God's kingdom. When we step into the family of God, we have the privilege of being part of His kingdom, and we also have the responsibility of upholding that kingdom. One of the ways we can do this is by staying close to God and sharing with other people what we have learned from our experiences (our "immunizations") so they can apply that knowledge and wisdom to their own lives and be protected from some of the anxiety and stresses they might otherwise have had. Just observing how a fellow believer responds to difficulties with trust in God, reflecting the life of Jesus, can strengthen people's faith. We uphold the kingdom by glorifying God and living the way of Jesus together with others in love and community. This community of love and care draws other people to God.

The early church grew quickly because people saw the fellowship that was happening among the believers. They saw their joy and their mutual love, respect, and sacrificial care. This type of lifestyle was rare in the Roman-occupied world, where people lied and cheated, and where Christians who did not recognize the Roman gods were persecuted and even put to death. But Jesus had made such a difference in the lives of His followers that they continued in His way despite the dangers and ridicule.

When we uphold the way of Jesus, it impacts our lives and the lives of everyone around us. And when, as a group, we're "chasing after Jesus" together and living for Him, it can prevent even the weakest of believers from leaving the path. There is power in following Christ in community—and danger in going our own way, doing our own thing. The danger is there for us *and* those around us.

When we stay inside the kingdom, we allow God to continue to do a work in us. It doesn't happen overnight, and again, it's not pixie dust, but God does steadily refine us to reflect more of Him. And while He works on us, we work on us, too. Philippians 2:12 reads, *"Continue to work out your salvation with fear and trembling."*

If a faith leader you greatly respect was encouraging you to work on your faith, you'd probably take it seriously. You'd be excited to have that person's focus and attention. You'd feel honored that they were willing to speak into your life, sharing their experience and wisdom. You'd probably feel a bit eager to make them proud—and maybe even a little worried that you'd do something to let them down. All of these feelings capture what I imagine it's like to work on something *"with fear and trembling."*

Jesus wants us to take our faith and our walk with Him seriously because we are His witnesses. (See Acts 1:8.) We are living examples of His work in human lives. We are testaments to His way of doing life. Working out this calling should make us intentional about not missing all that He has for us, and it should also have us trembling with excitement for what we *have* received. We can be "fearful" in a constructive way that takes our growth in God seriously while still freely functioning in peace and joy as we serve Him.

LIFE IN JESUS

As we began to talk about earlier, when we *"work out"* our salvation and our faith, and when we think about being refined and getting back to that garden-of-Eden relationship with God, sometimes we gauge our success by how things are going in life. We assume that if we're doing life well, we will produce a lot of fruit. While that perspective isn't entirely wrong, it's certainly misguided. Yes, working on our faith and our relationship with Jesus will produce fruit, but we must keep in mind that this kind of fruit doesn't come by striving or doing certain things or saying certain things. It has nothing to do with worldly measures of success. This kind of fruit comes solely from abiding in Jesus. (See John 15:4–5.)

In His Sermon on the Mount, recorded in Matthew 5–7, Jesus showed us what a life abiding in Him looks like. We often read those verses and nod our heads in agreement. Yes, we should be humbler; yes, we should be more others-minded. But if we are honest about what Jesus said, then we will also feel the incredible pressure of how impossible it can be to live in that way. Looking at those verses, we realize there is no way that we will ever measure up to them. There is no way that we can do what Jesus is asking us to do. The bar is set way too high.

But Jesus isn't asking us for perfection, and He certainly isn't asking us to figure this out on our own. He wants a relationship with us. He wants us to abide in Him so that He can give us the ability to tackle some things that we would never be able to overcome on our own.

True Spirit fruit happens when abiding happens. Resting in Jesus, relying on Him, seeking Him first, and practicing what are called "spiritual disciplines," such as reading God's Word, praying daily, fellowshipping regularly with other believers, fasting, giving, and solitude—we're not meant to do these things so that we can earn God's blessing but so that we can *learn* about His blessing. From this posture come the fruit and evidence of God's work in our lives.

I (Ronnie) used to have an orchard, and my plum trees were just incredible. The fruit was always sweet and healthy. The trees produced season after season, but not once did I hear them complain. The trees just sat there in the sun and soaked up the water and the nutrients I provided, and all of a sudden little flowers were growing on them. The flowers were always a sight to see, but it wasn't long before they'd die off, and the trees went back to looking like regular trees. You'd never know that those trees were working on something big. From the spots where those flowers had been came small green orbs that grew and grew and ripened, and by the end of the season, each orb had become a big, red, juicy plum.

The small green orbs were just as much plums as the large fruit were. It was all part of the process of growth. They were being the best plums they could be at the time. All they had to do was hang on and trust the tree to provide everything they needed to grow and mature into the plums they were meant to be.

That's what God wants to do with you. He wants you to rest in Him, to allow Him to nourish and feed you. To care for you and help you. And, over time, you'll change. It might not be noticeable at first. Or you might change in a big way only to realize that you still have far to go. But God longs to be with you. He actually wants more for you than you want for yourself.

When God's fruit starts coming alive in you, you'll realize that you're more at ease. You'll start to notice and be concerned for the people around you, not just yourself. You'll find that the things that made you angry don't bother you as much. You'll find yourself wanting to spend time in God's Word. You'll pray more. And, maybe for the first time in your life, you'll start to see just how much God loves you.

ANSWER HIS CALL

I (Ronnie) often laugh at the behavior of my ten grandchildren when they are playing together and something goes wrong. When a window breaks or someone gets hurt, I never have to ask, "Who did it?" I always know—it's the kid who isn't there. The other nine will be right there with me, helping to make things right, while the tenth—the one who made the mistake to begin with—is hiding.

Remember that this is what Adam and Eve did when they ate the fruit—they hid from God instead of going to Him to fix the problem.

But He did not let them stay hidden. He went looking for them. And, again, that's what He does with us—He comes looking for us! We are all inclined, because of our sin and shame, to distance ourselves from the One who makes things right. But Jesus has restored the path to rightness.

When was the last time you answered when God came looking for you? When was the last time you moved closer to community, trusting God when He said that it's not good for us to be alone? When was the last time you dug into His Word, made space for prayer, and truly abided in Him instead of relying on your intellect or fears to direct your path?

Distancing yourself from God and others only brings more feelings of shame, inadequacy, anxiety, and depression. It's time to turn toward Christ and abide in Him. He is the only path to true wholeness.

When we walk through our Anxiety Algorithm in more depth in part 2, we'll provide a model that will help you abide in Christ. But, for now, spend some time in prayer or sit in silence. Listen for His voice. Think upon His promises. Those are simple steps you can take today to abide in the One who longs to be with you.

WELLNESS EXERCISE: SCRIPTURE VISUALIZATION

Visualization is a technique that can be helpful in various ways in your Christian walk. It can be an aid for stress reduction, more meaningful prayer times, more intentional interaction with Scripture, and Scripture memorization.

This exercise is in the tradition of Christian meditation practices. Visualization is simply taking what you read and using your imagination to picture a scene or landscape in your mind. Using this technique can be very helpful because it engages the part of your brain associated with vision in order to create an image. This image helps you "see" what you are reading. We are not trying to change what the text says; we are simply improvising images and feelings as we read the passage to create a more real experience of the text. Any time you can engage more sensory information, whether by seeing, hearing, smelling, touching, or tasting, you are more likely to have a more meaningful experience. This also creates a more intense memory.

Try to use visualization to help you memorize Psalm 143:8–10. (We will focus on Scripture memorization further in the next wellness exercise.) It's always helpful to me (James) if I read a portion of a passage and then close my eyes and "see" the phrase before reading more. I will lead you through an example of how you might visualize this passage, but feel free to change the images to make it more applicable to you.

PSALM 143:8–10

Let the morning bring me word of your unfailing love....　　　(verse 8)

Imagine a beautiful morning. It may be in your favorite spot in your home, at the beach, in the mountains, or any other place that feels good and familiar. You may want to visualize God's "word of unfailing love" as a sunrise or the word "love" floating in the air toward you. The sunrise could represent a reminder of God's love for you, or the word "love" floating toward you would be a more literal image.

...for I have put my trust in you.　　　(verse 8)

Think about what trust looks like. A common way people think of faith and trust is that it is like sitting down in a chair and feeling secure that the chair will hold you. You may imagine sitting in God's lap or holding your hands out toward God like you are offering yourself to Him.

Show me the way I should go....　　　(verse 8)

Create a scene where you and Jesus begin to take a walk. Imagine His kind and compassionate face as He guides you along the path. You are not sure where He is taking you, but not knowing does not bother you because you are with Him on the journey.

...for to you I entrust my life.　　　(verse 8)

Let Jesus's kind and wise face create a feeling of full surrender and trust in your heart. This image can lead you to a place of total trust in Him and the thought that no one could ever make you feel more safe and secure.

> *Rescue me from my enemies,* LORD.... (verse 9)

As you walk down this road with Jesus, imagine that others come to rob you. Jesus simply says, "Stop," and they are unable to move. You feel amazed by how powerful Jesus's words are and how safe you feel with Him.

> *...for I hide myself in you.* (verse 9)

Jesus reaches out and embraces you, and it feels as if a gentle giant is hugging you. His arms totally envelop you, and you feel comforted and warm. You notice how good Jesus's garment smells as you hug Him. You don't want to stop hugging Him.

> *Teach me to do your will....* (verse 10)

As you continue walking with Jesus, you ask Him to teach you what you should do. He reassures you that He will never leave you, and that He will always guide you. He tells you that your job is to simply stay with Him as you journey. Again, you feel reassured and thankful.

> *...for you are my God....* (verse 10)

Along the road, you meet an old friend, and you introduce Jesus to them. You tell them that Jesus is your Savior and the kindest, wisest, and most noble person you have ever known. Jesus expresses to them how much He loves you and how much you mean to Him.

> *...may your good Spirit lead me on level ground.* (verse 10)

As you continue walking with Jesus, you realize He is not taking certain alternate paths that you pass from time to time. You ask Him why He is taking the path He has chosen. He explains that other paths have dangers you cannot see, and that the path He has chosen has shade and water nearby. He tells you that the path you are on also gives Him more time alone with you before you reach your destination and the busy city. His words bring you comfort, and you feel grateful for the beautiful morning and your walk with Jesus. You feel so loved that you want your walk with Jesus to continue forever.

Again, this is one example of many different ways you might visualize this passage. Hopefully, this was a meaningful experience for you. Visualization may be something you already do often, though perhaps without realizing it, and so the exercise may have felt more natural to you. Or, the experience may have felt strange and awkward for you. Either feeling is okay. The important thing is to take time to do the exercise so that you become more comfortable with it as you slow down and take in the words of the psalm.

9

GIVING OURSELVES TO GOD

I (Ronnie) had a friend in college who could play the guitar incredibly well. I remember being a little jealous and telling him that I wished I had the gift to play the way he did. I'll never forget the way he looked at me when I said that. He replied, "This isn't a gift, Ronnie. I practice all the time. I put in hours and hours—probably eight hours a day."

Realizing my mistake, I quickly apologized, but that exchange has stuck with me over the years. It reveals a lot about how we approach life, especially our spiritual lives.

Every single follower of Christ can have a deep, meaningful spiritual walk with Him. Every single one of us can have communion with God, hear His voice, have a sensitivity to the Spirit's promptings, and more. All we have to do is put in the time and effort.

Many of us, however, think that drastic change in our lives should happen over the course of a few days or weeks—not the years that it typically can take to develop a deep relationship with God. The things that truly matter in life aren't handed to us simply because we decide we want them. Again, they require a lot of work and a lot of time.

We often wait for God to do miracles because miracles don't require any effort on our part. We simply have to sit back and see what happens—and, if nothing happens, we shrug and think, "Maybe next time!"

But who wants to wait for a possible miracle when we can put into practice what will surely bring a response from God? Why wait when we can be building toward renewal and a complete change in our lives?

God honors us when we put forth the effort. When we do our part, then we get to see God do His. We get to see Him bring results that we couldn't have imagined were possible.

Picture a teenage daughter who loves to sew and who asks her parents for a sewing machine for Christmas. They give her a beautiful, top-of-the-line machine, and she receives it with joy, but the only thing she does with it is put it on a table and admire it. Weeks go by, and the daughter never actually uses the machine for sewing, saying she might do that "someday." Her parents ask, "Why did you ask for a sewing machine if you're never going to sew anything with it?"

It is a similar idea with our salvation. God didn't offer us a new life and hope in Him so that we could merely admire it or think about how one day we might fully enter into His gift. He gave us salvation so that we can "work it out"! Not to work *for* it but to allow it to change and teach us, resulting in our being able to release our anxiety and be made whole—all so that our lives can be fully transformed, we can make a difference in the world, and the people around us can see the power of the gospel in action.

But what does this actually look like? How do we fully "work out" our salvation?

A LIFESTYLE THAT LEADS TO WHOLENESS

We've talked a bit about this, but there is a method that we've found to be key to shifting your mindset from "displaying your salvation on a table" (where you might talk about wanting a deeper relationship with God but don't do anything about it) to putting in the work that will make your salvation come alive—which will also enable you to better address your anxiety. It's the difference between thinking about learning to play the guitar and putting in the practice to become the type of guitarist who blows everyone away by their commitment, passion, and skill.

It all comes down to Jesus's words from the passage in Mark 12 that we began to discuss in chapter 2. It's about giving God your heart, soul, mind, and strength. Once we understand that we don't need to hide from God, and we begin to move toward Him and His love, we can increasingly give over to Him every area of our lives for healing and restoration.

When Jesus was asked by a teacher of the law what the greatest commandment is, this was His response:

> "The most important one," answered Jesus, "is this: 'Hear, O Israel: The Lord our God, the Lord is one. Love the Lord your God with all your heart and with all your soul and with all your mind and with all your strength.' The second is this: 'Love your neighbor as yourself.' There is no commandment greater than these." (Mark 12:29–31)

If Jesus thought this was the best, most important commandment, then we ought to take it seriously and get to the bottom of what He was saying. To do this, we're going to spend a little time looking at what it means to give God our heart, soul, mind, and strength. Though it's hard to separate these areas from one another because they are so interconnected in who we are, for the sake of clarity, we're going to look at each part individually, and we're going to go from the bottom of the list to the top, starting with strength.

But before we explore this topic in greater depth in the next two chapters, it's important that we form a basic understanding of these four parts of ourselves:

1. *Strength.* This refers to our actions, what we do. These are the things that the outside world sees—the physical and external aspects of our lives.

2. *Mind.* The mind is the part of us that thinks and then controls or determines our actions. This aspect may seem straightforward, but that isn't always the case, a reality we will dive into later.

3. *Soul.* The soul (also often referred to as the "spirit") is the spiritual part of us, the part that is connected to God. Genesis 2:7 is a beautiful verse that says, *"Then the LORD God formed a man from the dust of the ground and breathed into his nostrils the breath of life, and the man became a living being."* Some translations say that man became a "living soul." It is through our soul that we communicate with God.

4. *Heart.* The heart refers to our emotions, our feelings.

These components are integral to who we are and how we connect with God and the world around us. But remember: Satan always takes what God intends for our good and tries to use it to separate us from God and prevent us from living in a way that is aware of His presence. Satan wants us to feel alone, to feel disconnected from the One who loves us. He wants us to stay in hiding, like Adam and Eve.

But God designed us to want to move toward wellness, *and* He is working everything out for His glory. To get a glimpse of what God is up to in this way, let's return to the story of Joseph. Joseph's brothers believed the lie that he was a threat (remember our discussion of perceived and actual threats?) and needed to be eliminated so that they could protect their own futures. (See Genesis 37:1–28.) But God took their broken, misled actions and used them for His glory.

All of the hard and difficult and ugly things in Joseph's life resulted in God's greatest blessings toward him and his family.

God is working things out for our good because He loves us.

Psalm 139 expresses this very love. In this psalm, David writes about how he is known by God—and the same applies to us. Nothing about you was a mistake. Satan wants you to feel as though you're so messed up and anxious that there's no way God can help you, let alone love you. He wants you to believe that there is no way you can overcome your weaknesses, your inadequacies, your failures, your errors, the sin in your life. But the truth is that God can fix anything that needs to be fixed. He can make beauty from pain and darkness, and because of this, it's important to open yourself up to the possibility that things can be made right.

Just consider that for a moment. Your anxiety, your fear, your worry—they can be made right.

In the next two chapters, we'll take a closer look at how this occurs as we unpack each of the means through which we love God and follow God—our strength, mind, soul, and heart.

10

UNPACKING OUR STRENGTH AND MIND

What is the nature of our strength—the physical side of us and our actions?

THE NATURE OF OUR STRENGTH

There are two kinds of actions: intentional and reflexive.[21] An example of this is how we learn simple math. At first, we have to work very hard at mastering the multiplication tables. We go over and over them, working them out. Yet, in time, we know the answers without having to think about them. We respond reflexively instead of having to spend time intentionally doing the math in our heads.

The same is true of the process of learning to read. Grace is my (Ronnie's) youngest child. When she packed for college, my wife and I were helping her clean out her closet, and I found an old stack of index cards with a single word written on each of them. Grace didn't remember them, but we had used those cards to go over her sight

---

21. Dr. Anthony Huberman, "How to Focus to Change Your Brain," Huberman Lab podcast, February 8, 2021, 1:25:15, https://www.youtube.com/watch?app=desktop&v=LG53Vxum0as.

words with her every day while she waited for the school bus. She spent all of that time intentionally learning those words, and now she's a college grad who can read and talk and text and watch her kids play all at the same time!

When we spend time practicing our faith and our love for God, we begin to move those areas from being intentional actions to reflexive actions. This is absolutely life-changing when it happens, because when loving God is reflexive, everything gets easier. You don't have to think as much about whether or not to do the "right thing." You won't experience days when God is the furthest thing from your mind while you're just trying to survive. When love and truth and peace constitute your natural state in Christ, then that is the position from which you will move through life. You may face failure or hardship, but when your actions are rooted in the presence of God and are reflective of His qualities, life gets a whole lot easier.

As we practice remaining in God's presence, then when things happen that push us away from God, we will reflexively step back toward Him and His presence instead of moving further away from Him. But for that to happen—for us to love God with our actions—we must spend a lot of time taking intentional steps. We must put in the work.

Again, that's what the Anxiety Algorithm is all about and what these beginning chapters are designed to prepare you to do: move into a keen awareness of God's presence in your life. So much so that, over time, remaining with Him will become the norm and not the exception for you.

In my (Ronnie's) pediatric practice, ninth graders would come for their yearly checkup, and we'd inevitably talk about how they were struggling with algebra. I'd ask them one question: "What is seven times eight?" They'd pause for too long and then spit out 59 or 56, and I would show them that it wasn't algebra that they were struggling with—it was the basic math facts that had not yet become reflexive for them. My reasoning was that if they were still spending intentional energy on multiplication, how could they possibly master algebra?

Similarly, we need to learn to be reflexive in our spiritual responses because Satan works fast. So fast that we can't afford to be working out the basic math of our relationship with God every time things get hard. We have to be reflexive so that when stressors or crises happen, we're already in the presence of God without having to think about it.

Of course, God is with us all the time; His presence is all around us. In fact, He lives within us. But when we haven't learned to be reflexive, we aren't aware of Him. When we aren't aware of Him, we jump back into reacting to life from a worldly perspective that is focused on us and our wants and needs, our fears and stressors, rather than on God.

It takes time for a reflexive lifestyle to become habit, but God is patient with us.

When children are learning to walk, they stumble and fall. They have to strengthen their legs and their core muscles, and they have to get their balance figured out. It can take months or more for them to go from crawlers to confident walkers.

During this process, their parents cheer them on. They encourage them and help them to improve—and they get excited because their children are developing reflexive life skills. God is the same with us. He is glorified when we are putting in the intentional work of learning to abide in His presence. When we fall down, He is there to pick us back up and to remind us of *whose* we are and who He created us to be. Then He reminds us to keep our eyes on Him as we continue to intentionally learn how to walk in His presence. Just like a loving parent, He knows we are going to fall—falling is part of learning. His arms are outstretched, beckoning us to continue to work, strive, and press on to get closer and closer to Him.

Life is often about practicing things that initially might be very hard for us to do until we've spent time doing them and mastered them—and we should expect our relationship with God to be no different.

THE NATURE OF OUR MIND

We will face circumstances or stumbling blocks that have the potential to throw us off course and put to the test everything that we've been working on in our relationship with God. Such encounters can be jarring and unpleasant, but let us tell you something: your mind *can* handle them. And a mind that has God-centered clarity in times of danger or frustration or hardship is a mind that loves God.

When you experience unexpected physical danger, such as coming upon a snake in the grass, your brain immediately floods itself with the hormone epinephrine. This lights up your whole brain and body, putting you on full alert. Your heart will start racing, your breath will quicken, and you'll start trembling and sweating. All of this happens as your body waits for your next move.

Additionally, while epinephrine turns on the big lights in your body, the neurotransmitter acetylcholine turns on the spotlight. This spotlight zeros in on the danger and tells you not to run toward the snake. It tells you to get away from it. It helps you to find a path toward safety.

The longer these chemicals need to shine a light on the danger, the faster you'll wear out and become stressed. But the sooner you can develop your path of escape, the calmer you'll remain. This is why chronic stress (which we talked about earlier and will discuss further in a coming chapter) is so detrimental.

Most of the time, the path toward safety involves using the Two Steps Back method we discussed in chapter 6. It involves distancing yourself from the danger without turning your back on it completely. Once you do this, the neurotransmitter dopamine charges in, encouraging you that you're on the right path. Dopamine keeps you going, and once you are safe from danger, serotonin rushes in to tell you that you are safe, to give you peace. At this point, your heart rate will come down, and your breathing will calm. You might be trembling a bit from the adrenaline rush, but your body is recovering from survival mode.

Too much of any of these chemicals is not a good thing, but, together, they do a great job of keeping us levelheaded and protected. God created us in this way. He created these chemicals to work together so that we can think clearly in dangerous situations and make the best decisions going forward. Isn't it great that science is now explaining how God put us together so *"fearfully and wonderfully"* (Psalm 139:14)?

We love the way Dr. Judy Willis, in an article for *Psychology Today* online, explained the way our brains work:

> Neuroplasticity [the fact that the brain changes] is the process through which thoughts, experiences, and actions transform the brain. This ability of the brain to change evolves across our entire lifetimes. The way it works is that each time a memory circuit activates (used, remembered, applied), electric impulses travel through it. These impulses generate more expansive and stronger connections (synapses, dendrites, myelin coating axons) among the brain cells (neurons) of that memory circuit. The newly enhanced information becomes more durable, more readily retrieved, and more easily applied to new applications....
>
> ...*This means that with practice and effort we can build the brains we want.*[22]

Of course, neuroplasticity is at its best when we're younger—a child can learn a new language faster than an adult can—but our brains are still changing and learning even when we're older. Electric impulses travel through the brain via neurons. Billions of these neurons tell your brain to eat, sleep, walk, and more. They come together and communicate with one another in what are called synapses, and that's where these neurons become pathways. Our brains form these pathways, and they can develop what we refer to as "ruts," where the neurons tend to travel the same paths over and over. Now, the word *rut* can be thought of as

---

22. Judy Willis, MD, MEd, "Memory: How Practice Makes Permanent," *Psychology Today*, June 22, 2018, https://www.psychologytoday.com/us/blog/radical-teaching/201806/memory-how-practice-makes-permanent. Emphasis added.

describing something negative, and, in some cases, it may be. But in the case of good habit formation, such ruts or pathways are a good thing! They are part of the process of how something goes from being intentional to being reflexive, or from taking great effort to taking little effort. Or, to use our earlier example of a toddler, from falling a lot to walking without even thinking about it. We must realize that it takes work to break out of a rut that has been leading to a bad outcome. It takes intentionality to do things differently, to open yourself to a new way of thinking or living—to a new ingrained pathway—but it's definitely possible.

The things that you do over and over again (the things you put into practice) become information that is more reflective to you; you can more readily retrieve it and more easily apply it. The positive actions that you put into practice when you're in a high-stress situation can be the same actions that you do reflexively while just walking through life. Once you groove that new neural pathway, you can use it over and over, whether you're in a high-risk situation or a low-risk one.[23]

With practice and effort, we can build the brains—the lives— that we want. This is how God made us!

One way we can do this is by becoming memorizers of Scripture. We can also practice abiding in Christ every moment of our day. We can allow Him to produce the fruit of His Spirit in us: *"Love, joy, peace, patience, kindness, goodness, faithfulness, gentleness, self-control"* (Galatians 5:22–23 ESV). This fruit not only makes our lives better but also positively affects the lives of those around us.

When we build the brains and lives we want, we can tackle anxiety and stressors with calm clarity as we sit in the presence of God. This has nothing to do with how smart, how spiritual, or how gifted we are. Again, it has everything to do with our *intention* to put in the work. We can all change with practice and effort as we train our minds to be focused on Christ. This is how we love God with all of our mind, and this is how we move toward wellness.

---

23. Dr. Anthony Huberman, "How Your Nervous System Works and Changes," Huberman Lab podcast, January 4, 2021, 36:25, https://www.youtube.com/watch?v=H-XfCl-HpRM.

11

UNPACKING OUR SOUL AND HEART

Paul wrote, *"Those who live in accordance with the Spirit have their minds set on what the Spirit desires"* (Romans 8:5). This shift away from pursuing what we want apart from God to what the Spirit wants might feel like a huge sacrifice at first, but the reward is peace. A soul in tune with the Spirit has peace.

THE NATURE OF THE SOUL

Loving God with our soul starts with salvation. It's very hard to live a Christian life and depend on God if you don't have a relationship with Him through the person of His Son, Jesus. So if you have never come to a place in your life where you've relinquished control and turned it all over to Him, that is step one.

Loving God with our soul also means setting aside the kingdoms that we want to build so that we can make room for what God is building. A soul in tune with the Lord is intentional about reading and studying the Bible and praying in order to better understand God and what He desires. That soul loves Jesus and seeks to know Him intimately, not just as words on a page but as an active part of their life.

This isn't a matter of working toward our salvation but rather working *because* of it. It's not about earning the love of God—it's about having the love of God in us and what that means for the world around us.

Our soul allows us to love and follow God by shedding the parts of us that strive for His favor, replacing them with a pure openness to Him and His kingdom. Yes, we are sinful; yes, we are fallen; but our soul isn't concerned as much with what we've done than with who we are becoming. It allows us to experience God's presence in the here and now, even with all of the baggage we carry. When we allow that to happen, when we open ourselves up to receiving God's love and grace, in spite of our shortcomings, that is a true act of love toward God. That is loving Him with all our soul.

THE NATURE OF THE HEART

Our emotions—the feelings we have—are real and very important. But they can absolutely get in the way of loving and following Christ.

Frustration, guilt, anxiety, and shame due to our mistakes and failures: as we have seen, these feelings can contribute to a fixed mindset that gets us to believe we are incapable of change, are inherently bad, or can't be helped.

When people have this mindset, it results in their pulling away from God because they have determined that they can't measure up and that they will only disappoint God, those around them, and, ultimately, themselves.

This state of mind is so far from where God wants us to be! The only way out of it is to become intentional about changing your mindset and learning how to control your emotions and debilitating thoughts rather than letting them control you.

Every single promise found in the Bible is available to you. Every single one. No, we don't deserve this, but that's why God's promises are given to us *"in Christ"* (2 Corinthians 1:20). It's through Him that we are able to receive what God wants to give us.

A. W. Tozer said, "God wills that we should push on into his presence and live our whole life there."[24] Our emotions will tell us to give up, but God wants us to stay with Him, to keep our heart, our emotions, in His presence. We were not made to handle our emotions on our own. From the beginning, God's plan was to be right there with us, helping us work through our feelings to find truth, hope, and light. But His contribution will get buried if we aren't also doing our part.

When Jesus came up out of the water after being baptized, the Spirit came upon Him. Luke tells us that, immediately after this, *"Jesus, full of the Holy Spirit, left the Jordan and was led by the Spirit into the wilderness, where for forty days he was tempted by the devil. He ate nothing during those days, and at the end of them he was hungry"* (Luke 4:1–2).

This passage blew me (Ronnie) away when I sat down to really study it. The idea that the Spirit led Jesus into the wilderness so that He would be tempted was beyond confusing to me. That must have been very stressful for Jesus, but He resisted Satan by relying on and quoting Scripture He had memorized. After that, *"Jesus returned to Galilee in the power of the Spirit, and news about him spread through the whole countryside"* (verse 14).

The stressful and emotional situations Jesus experienced during His time in the wilderness prepared Him for His ministry, because even He needed to allow the power of the Spirit to rule over His emotions and desires. As He responded to those temptations in a reflexive way from all the preparations He had made through prayer and reading the Scriptures as a boy and as a young man, Jesus experienced the limitless power that was within Him. And we are told in Ephesians 1:19–21 that the same power that raised Jesus from the dead is available to us.

Giving our emotions and desires to Jesus and relying on His Spirit to get us through—that is what it means to love God with our whole heart.

---

24. A. W. Tozer, *The Pursuit of God: The Human Thirst for the Divine* (Harrisburg, PA: Christian Publications Incorporated, 1948), 24.

THE INTERACTION BETWEEN HEART AND MIND

Now that we've reviewed the four means through which we express our love for God—strength, mind, soul, and heart—let's look a little more closely at the interaction between our heart and our mind. Your mind (your thoughts) controls your actions, but it also controls your emotions, as we talked about above. This is important, because some people let their emotions rule. Five-year-olds are great examples of this. One of my (Ronnie's) young grandsons was having trouble completing his memory verse, and he responded by complaining, whining, and crying—he had an emotional outburst because he was frustrated.

As we age, we all learn to have some control over our emotions, yet many of us, when our backs are against the wall, let our emotions call the shots. When we come across a snake, instead of taking two steps back, we run around screaming!

We've talked previously about the biblical figure of Joseph, who shows us that it's truly possible to have control over our emotions. Instead of allowing the chemicals in him to take charge, Joseph was in charge of the chemicals. He stayed cool and calm when things around him were absolutely chaotic. And, at the very end, he was able to say that what others had intended for harm, God had intended for good. (See Genesis 50:15–20.) Now *that* is where we want to be!

This doesn't mean that we shouldn't ever get upset. Emotions are important; they are God-given to help us understand and process the world around us. It's good and right to become upset or fearful or sad or disappointed when the situation calls for it. *The key, though, is to not let that emotion determine your next step.* For example, you might be upset by the fact that your boss chose someone else for a promotion, but that doesn't mean that you should quit your job or lash out at a coworker.

Allowing our emotions to determine what we do next is often a sign that we don't believe that we will be taken care of. We don't believe that we are capable of finding a clear path out or through.

This approach to life can be developed in us during childhood. Parents who are quick to help or protect their child in situations where the child is not in any real danger end up communicating to their son or daughter that they are weak and incapable of doing things without their parents' help. This is how a parent's lack of emotional maturity can trickle down to their child. The parent sees the world as dangerous and scary, and so their actions of doing what they feel is protecting their child end up promoting the same mindset in them: that the world is scary, and that the child is weak and incapable.

A great example of this was when my (James's) wife, Jessica, and I brought our eighteen-month-old son Covington to visit Grandpa (Ronnie). We were all standing outside, and Covington was sitting on the ground eating dirt! Jessica and I noticed what was happening, and we looked at each another. (Meanwhile, my dad started laughing!) However, instead of freaking out and jumping into the situation, we looked over at Dad and asked, "Is that dangerous?"

He didn't think it was, and so we let Covington continue to explore the world around him without his loving parents getting in the way. If we had jumped in and made a big deal about what he was doing, it would have sent a message that dirt was bad for him. A few more instances of our promoting the idea that nature is "bad," and we might have ended up with a son who was afraid to explore the great outdoors! But because we kept calm and viewed the situation through a rational lens instead of an emotional lens, we were able to encourage Covington to get dirty and have fun. When we control our emotions, we clarify our mindset and allow ourselves and others to thrive.

Stanford professor and podcaster Alia Crum defines *mindset* as "your core beliefs or assumptions you make about a domain; your expectations, explanations, goals, and motivation."[25] We think that is a very accurate description of what constitutes our mindsets.

---

25. Dr. Alia Crum, "Science of Mindsets for Health & Performance," Huberman Lab podcast, Episode 56, January 24, 2022, 8:26, https://podcastnotes.org/huberman-lab/episode-56-dr-alia-crum-science-of-mindsets-for-health-performance-huberman-lab/.

There was a fascinating study in which people were divided into two groups and then given milkshakes. One group was told that the milkshakes were completely healthy, with no fats or sugars, but that the taste was mediocre. The other group was told that the milkshakes had extra fat and sugar but tasted great. In reality, the milkshakes were the same, but when the researchers tested the blood of the participants, they found that the group that had been told that their shakes was unhealthy were more satisfied. Chemicals in their blood that indicated satisfaction were more elevated after the milkshake—all because their mindset told them they would be satisfied. The group that had been told that their milkshakes were healthy but mediocre in taste were apparently less satisfied, since those chemicals were not as elevated in them. They had consumed their milkshakes with the mindset that it would not be a great experience for them, and so it wasn't, both mentally and physiologically![26] That is how powerful a mindset can be.

Your core beliefs are therefore the assumptions you make about a domain: your expectations—including about your milkshake!—explanations, goals, and motivation. When we approach a situation thinking that it's going to go well, then we usually come out more satisfied than when we approach a situation assuming the worst.

FOUR TYPES OF MINDSETS

There are many types of mindsets, but here we will focus on four that are particularly relevant to dealing with anxiety and stress. The first is the *fixed mindset*, which has to do with labels: "You're so smart." "You're so beautiful." "You're damaged." "You're incapable of change." People who have a fixed mindset handle their errors more emotionally.

Next, there is the *growth mindset*, which incorporates verbs and looks at the effort put in: "You tried so hard." "You really hung in there." "You really hustled out there." People with this mindset handle

---

26. Crum, "Science of Mindsets for Health & Performance," 14:45.

their errors more cognitively. They will think about their mistakes and adjust their behavior instead of reacting emotionally to them.

It has been shown that children perform better and handle life more easily when they have a growth mindset. When told that they are smart (fixed mindset), many children don't try as hard, whereas when praised for their effort (growth mindset), they blow everyone away with their subsequent accomplishments.

A fixed mindset keeps us afraid of failure. If we don't measure up, we're afraid of losing the label that we believe makes us special or of reinforcing a label of failure, so, many times, we don't even try. But a growth mindset keeps us learning. It gives us space to fail because we are not defined by results. We are defined by effort.[27]

Then there are stress mindsets. Someone with a *stress-can-be-enhancing mindset* focuses on handling a challenging situation, coming up with a solution, and getting better. They reason that stress can actually make them better, and so it does. On the other hand, someone with a *stress-is-debilitating mindset* says that all stress is bad, harmful, and should be avoided, no matter what.

With a *stress-can-be-enhancing* mindset, we see stress as a means to improve ourselves and grow, to learn how to tackle hard things. We love cutting new grooves in the brain, making new pathways that will affect our entire lives for the better.[28]

The age-old mentality of, "This is just the way I am; I can't do any better" scientifically does not fly anymore. The way we are is not the way we have to remain. In fact, the way we are doesn't even come close to determining our potential, because when we start to combine the growth mindset with the stress-can-be-enhancing mindset, we start to see breakthrough.

My (Ronnie's) friend's granddaughter is a golfer. My friend got to be with her during one of her tournaments, and he couldn't stop

---

27. Carol S. Dweck, PhD, *Mindset: The New Psychology of Success* (New York: Ballantine Books, 2016), 6–7, 16–17.
28. Crum, "Science of Mindsets for Health & Performance," 45:00.

talking to her about how talented she was. A few holes in, she began to get frustrated and down on herself. Things weren't going as well as she'd hoped, and the fun was gone. My friend realized what was happening, and he changed his approach because of what he had recently been learning about mindsets. Instead of telling his granddaughter how great she was at golf, he began to praise her for how hard she was working. He'd give her honest feedback about her putts and then praise her effort and tenacity.

The day turned around for her, and not only did she score very well, but she also had a great time doing it.

This story brings the growth mindset to life, and it's a glimpse at how God sees us. He's far more interested in our effort than in our performance, because He doesn't *need* us to achieve His will. He doesn't *need* us to perform a certain way for Him to be glorified. But what He wants is for us to give it all we've got.

My (Ronnie's) parents always praised my effort—and it might have been by default, because when I played football, I didn't have much talent! In my junior year, I was third-string center, destined to ride out the season on the bench.

However, the first-string center got hurt, and then the second-string center had to play defense, so the coaches put me into the game. You should have seen the looks on their faces! It was clear they didn't have much hope for me or for the team. But you'd better believe that I played as hard as I could. I put everything into my position on that team, and, by my senior year, I was starting center and team captain. I still am the only person that I know of in Pascagoula (Mississippi) High School football history to get most improved player two years in a row. Even someone with little athletic ability can continue to improve; I am proof of that.

We stress over the things that are most important to us. Alia Crumb explains it like this: if a student you don't know or with whom you have only an acquaintance is failing at school, that probably doesn't stress you out very much. But if that student is your child, suddenly you're very concerned, very invested, and very stressed.[29]

Life and relationships become stressful because we care. When things are not the way they're supposed to be—when they're not the way God intended them to be—it gets to us, drawing us in emotionally. In this situation, the appropriate mindset is to allow this stress to help us grow and make us better. To allow our concern and worry to push us to improve our relationships and life.

And we do this by approaching things differently so we can groove new paths. Instead of emphasizing what others are doing wrong, we begin to focus on how *we* can change and better honor God in our relationships. When we allow stress to transform us, we move from "I'm frustrated" to "How can I help?" Responding constructively when we encounter stress is a sign that we're making progress.

A primary message in this chapter is to avoid a performance-based mindset, but here's where it gets interesting. When you adopt a growth mindset and see stress as a way to improve your life and relationships, you become really good at analyzing performance. You become adept at seeing what works and what doesn't, and at accommodating to attain the best results.

This isn't because your worth is in your performance. It's because your worth is in your value to God and in who He created you to be. So, you want your effort to be the best it can be to produce the best results possible.

Ultimately, our goal should be to have the same mindset as Jesus, but for this to happen, we must open ourselves up to a bit of stress so that we can be refined and changed and improved. When we concentrate just on the mess of life around us, we'll be stressed in a bad way. But when we allow God to work through us, stress can be something that brings us closer to others, closer to Him, and more impactful in life.

---

29. Crum, "Science of Mindsets for Health & Performance."

WELLNESS EXERCISE: SCRIPTURE MEMORIZATION

One of the core building blocks to a growth mindset—and what we have found helps folks who struggle with anxiety and depression—is Scripture memorization.

We are all capable of memorizing Scripture. We may go at different paces, and some of us may have a goal of learning one verse per year, while others may be memorizing entire books of the Bible. Regardless of how much we are able to memorize, the thing that matters most is the time we put into it.

A few years ago, God challenged me (Ronnie) to make Scripture memorization a priority. I had always had a good prayer life, and I'd always read Scripture, but God was asking me to hide His Word in my heart. So, I took Him up on the challenge.

I told God that I would offer Him at least thirty minutes every day, to be devoted to memorizing Deuteronomy chapter 6. It took me six months to reach my goal—so it wasn't as if I was memorizing at breakneck speed! Slow and steady wins the race. But then God surprised me. I sensed Him asking me to memorize more Scripture. He wanted this to be a daily practice.

I began driving around with my Bible app on the audio setting, and I recited passages along with the narrator. Day after day, I made progress, and, more than that, I discovered that memorizing Scripture grounds me.

No other spiritual discipline has empowered me like Scripture memorization. I have found that it makes me more aware of God's presence moment by moment. His Word, by the power of His Spirit, comes into my mind throughout the day—it's really amazing. I will be going through life, thinking about regular things, and then a passage of Scripture will come up in my mind—the perfect passage for whatever situation I'm in.

Jesus quoted Scripture all the time—in particular, in the wilderness and on the cross, two of the most stressful times of His life. It makes sense that we should do the same.

Part Two:

APPLYING THE ANXIETY ALGORITHM

12

THE ALGORITHM PLAN

In chapter 2, we asked you to consider the question "What does it mean to be well?"—to think about what wellness looks like. As we begin to explore the algorithm, we want to ask you a similar question: "What would peace look like for you?" If you have extreme anxiety, you might not even know how to answer that question, but we encourage you to do your best. Write down what a life of peace might look like. Ask the Spirit to help you, and think about friends who exhibit peace in their lives. What are some things that you admire about the way they go about living? What are some beautiful things you see in their lives that you would love to have in your own life?

Write it all down, even the bits that you haven't fully figured out, and sign the paper as if you are handing it off to God. This is what your hope is for your life. But as you sign it off to God, tell Him that it's not your will but His will that you want more than anything. You may know from experience or from reading the Bible that as God works and moves, He will likely do something very different from what your vision is. But the special part about this is that His work will be perfectly tailored for you, and it will exceed anything you can ask or imagine. (See Ephesians 3:20.)

As you open your heart and mind to the possibility of God moving, He might impress names upon your heart—people who can walk with you and support you. He may also lead you into acts of service. Volunteering in the church nursery or using your talents at a local nonprofit—whatever prompting you receive, don't push it away. Our serving others is a way in which God gets a hold of us, and it very well could be part of His plan for healing us.

Whatever is impressed upon your heart, if it is in line with Scripture, then you know it's probably from God, and you can walk confidently forward, trusting that He will make your path straight. It is tempting to want to know every step of the way in advance, but if God were to reveal all the steps in this manner, we might not take that first step. We might even dread what's next, because this is not going to be an easy journey. That's why we must trust Him.

It's been said that people with anxiety live too much in the future, and people with depression live too much in the past. We must become people who live in the moment, relying on the Spirit for every good thing and being emotionally healthy to step into what is before us, letting the past be the past and leaving the future up to our King.

THE IMPACT OF SCRIPTURE

Learning to live in the moment, trusting in God, has completely changed my (Ronnie's) life. There was a time about twenty-five years ago when I was really struggling. I felt like I had absolutely no hope. Several things were causing excess stress in my life. One was my father's illness, and another was dealing with my medical practice. It seemed like life was spiraling out of control. My ability to function day-to-day was coming to a standstill. I didn't know how to keep on keeping on. One day, at work, I paused and gave it all over to God. I told Him that I had no hope or peace for my future, that all I felt was despair. I got back to work and opened my email, and a Bible devotion hit my inbox. At the top was Romans 15:13: *"May the God of hope fill you with all joy and peace as you trust in him, so that you may overflow with hope by the power of the Holy Spirit."* I had gone to God with my hopelessness, and He had showed up with a promise of hope from Scripture. I couldn't believe it.

I wrote Romans 15:13 on sticky notes and put them everywhere—in my bathroom, in my car, in my wallet. Then I memorized this verse and recited it every time I felt hopeless, and I went from experiencing total depression to bursting with joy and hope. It seems almost too good to be true, but it happened!

The promises of God work. His truth found in Scripture works. The Word of God is living and active, and it brings truth into our lives. We are promised that it *"judges the thoughts and attitudes of the heart"* (Hebrews 4:12). Jesus promised that if we follow Him and His teachings, then we *"will know the truth, and the truth will set [us] free"* (John 8:32)—and we believe this promise includes freedom from depression, anxiety, fear, and hopelessness.

Anxiety is an attack on our soul, and God longs to help us fight it. Again, one of the best weapons we have is Scripture. Jesus used Scripture to ward off Satan in the wilderness, and we can use it today to address whatever we're facing, whatever hopelessness has overcome us. We have a heavenly Father who knows what we're going through because He is already right here with us. He knows our struggles and our fears, and He longs to help us.

What Scripture do you need? What promise from God will change your life? What does God say about your situation and the way you feel? How does He want to move? The Anxiety Algorithm will help you learn to draw close to God through the truths of Scripture.

UNFOLDING THE ALGORITHM

The verses that changed my (Ronnie's) life and the life of my friend Shane so many years ago, from which James and I developed the Anxiety Algorithm, are Philippians 4:8–9:

> *Finally, brothers and sisters, whatever is true, whatever is noble, whatever is right, whatever is pure, whatever is lovely, whatever is admirable—if anything is excellent or praiseworthy—think about such things. Whatever you have learned or received or heard from me, or seen in me—put it into practice. And the God of peace will be with you.*

We found that this simple passage, when broken down and applied to one's life, can be an incredible tool for dealing with stress and anxiety. This passage helped us bring our focus back to Christ; and, over time, that intentionality became so reflexive that many of the anxious thoughts and worries we had experienced were completely gone.

It's important to reemphasize here that the Anxiety Algorithm is not a replacement for medication or therapy. Those tools are essential for many people living with depression and extreme anxiety, and, many times, they can be helpful for people who are fearful or anxious. Talk therapy is beneficial, whether you struggle with anxious thoughts or not! So, in no way is this approach a replacement for those traditional methods. Instead, it should be viewed as another tool in the toolbox, with the hope that as time goes on, it will become more and more valuable and effective for you.

An Invitation to the God of Peace

Let's review the definition of an algorithm: "a step-by-step procedure for solving a problem or accomplishing some end." As we wrote at the beginning of this book, an algorithm is a plan. More than just a solution to a problem, an algorithm can also create a lot of good, making something beautiful out of something that is broken. As you walk through the passage from Philippians 4, you can learn to quiet your anxiety and experience peace instead.

What makes this algorithm a unique tool is that it's a way to invite the God of peace into your life, and it is a focused effort to experience His presence more tangibly. This goes beyond chasing an emotion or trying to regulate your body so that you feel a certain way. This is about inviting the person of God to make Himself more known to you in the here and now. The goal of the algorithm is more of Him in your life.

Near the end of His earthly life, Jesus was under incredible stress. He knew what God was calling Him to do, but instead of getting angry at His disciples or getting so drunk that He wouldn't have to deal with it, Jesus went straight to His Father. He spent the night before His crucifixion praying in the garden of Gethsemane. In this prayer, He confessed His feelings and mindset. He begged God to change His mind, to make another way to save humanity. He asked for help in dealing with what probably felt like an impossible task—knowingly entering into torture and death is not something anyone would feel confident about! During His prayer, He experienced psychological symptoms of stress that were so intense that He was ministered to by an angel. (See, for example, Luke 22:41–44.)

Yet, ultimately, Jesus put it all into God's hands. He accepted what was before Him and relied on His relationship and trust with the Father to move forward even when He was scared and stressed. He found comfort in the presence of God, so much so that He was able to set aside His fear and anxiety, and take up the cross.

Following the Focal Points

We can receive and experience the presence of God in much the same way Jesus did, and, again, the passage in Philippians 4 is a great tool to lead us into that mindset. By going through each of the focal points in the passage, we can (1) settle our minds, (2) quiet the noise, (3) guide our thoughts, and (4) receive the presence of God in our lives—similar to what we described with the Two Steps Back method, which helps us to become established in this practice. The focal points are the following:

- Thinking about something that is true.
- Thinking about something that is noble.

- Thinking about something that is right.
- Thinking about something that is pure.
- Thinking about something that is lovely.
- Thinking about something that is admirable.
- Thinking about something that is excellent.
- Thinking about something that is praiseworthy.

Each of the focal points is somewhat specific and direct, but while there may be some overlap, the way that you think about them or approach them will be very different from the way your spouse or friend thinks about them or approaches them. There is freedom and flexibility to make this plan what you need it to be so that you can quickly and honestly shift your mindset from one of worry to one of peace.

Once more, the idea behind the algorithm is that whenever you need a mindset of peace, you can move through each of the focal points, first thinking about something that is true, then something that is noble, and so on down the list until you feel the peaceful presence of God in a way that you hadn't felt when you were getting lost in your fear and stress. In times of high anxiety, you may need to walk through the algorithm a dozen times before you begin to feel it work; but, over time, you will find that you won't even reach the end of the focal points before you feel the powerful and comforting presence of Jesus. The intentional will become reflexive.

Because the algorithm can be tailored to what is most meaningful to you, it might be helpful to ask the Spirit to guide you as you go through each of the focal points. Ask Him to identify which image would be best for you to focus on while you are meditating there: An image of your family? A memory? A Scripture verse? A Bible story? You can try different ones until you land on something that works for you.

Our hope is that the algorithm will be something that you can use in an ongoing way to move out of an emotional response to a situation and into the knowledge that the God of peace is with you all the time.

It's important to note that the algorithm, in and of itself, doesn't bring God into your life. The passage from Philippians doesn't open a door that is usually closed. God is with us all the time. Even now, even in your darkest, most anxious moments, He is there, and His presence indwells you. But being aware of that presence is another thing entirely. The algorithm helps with awareness.

Meditation has gotten a bad reputation in some Christian circles, but we know from research that when it is approached in a healthy way—such as in the case of scripturally based reflection—it has positive effects on the brain. A simple definition of meditation is being very intentional about what you choose to focus your thoughts on. While some forms of meditation encourage the emptying of the mind and the removal of all thought, spiritual meditation practices focus on holy thoughts that are relevant to the moment—and that is the type of meditation that the algorithm encourages.

Spiritual mediation is a great way to focus on Scripture, and that's why we use meditation to help us concentrate on the focal points in Philippians 4:8. By thinking or meditating upon things that are true, noble, right, and so on, we are able to personalize these words and apply them directly to whatever we are facing or struggling with. While you are meditating, random thoughts will certainly pop in and try to steal the show—it's almost certain that you'll suddenly remember something that you need to add to the grocery list or a task that you had previously forgotten about—but being mindful of these distractions and setting them aside or writing them down to address later are great ways to keep your mind where you want it.

Spiritual meditation takes practice, and the more you work at it, the better you will become at allowing the right thoughts in and reorienting your mind to focus on them. Even Paul knew this would be the case when, in Philippians 4:9, he said to *"put it into **practice**."*

In the next chapter, we explain in more depth how to personalize the algorithm for the most helpful results.

13

PERSONALIZING THE ALGORITHM

It's possible that you could approach the Anxiety Algorithm in a very in-the-moment way and just wing it when it comes to thinking about things that are true, noble, right, pure, lovely, admirable, excellent, and praiseworthy. But the more personal you are with your thoughts, the more effective the experience will be. And to be personal with your thoughts, you'll need to put some effort into connecting with each of the focal points in a way that is very true and powerful for *you*.

As you look at a focal point, try to think of what it means to you. Imagine visuals or experiences that bring the word or concept to life in a way that gives you spiritual peace or a desire for peace. We'll shortly share some examples of things that you might think about for each of the focal points, but there are no right or wrong answers. What is noble to you may not signify nobleness to another; what is lovely for someone else may not seem lovely to you. The impact and effectiveness will be different. So, again, there is room to adapt the algorithm to your life and your experiences. As long as your focal point is Spirit-filled and positive and impactful, it's right for the algorithm.

As you build your storehouse of holy things to think about, you will find that you have a tool to use whenever anxiety hits. Whether you're at work or school, in a high-stress meeting, or at a doctor's appointment that has you on edge, you'll be able to move through each of the focal points and open yourself up to feeling God's presence more fully, which will bring His peace.

Let's now walk through the different focal points and discuss what they might look like.

WHATEVER IS TRUE

> *To the Jews who had believed him, Jesus said, "If you hold to my teaching, you are really my disciples. Then you will know the truth, and the truth will set you free."* (John 8:31–32)

Satan has lies that he loves to tell us, and those lies contribute to our anxiety in a big way. One of the best ways to counter them is with truth—the truth of who God is and of His relationship to us. Countering lies with truth does not come naturally when we have developed a pattern of listening to those lies. But the struggle to make focusing on the truth reflexive is absolutely worth it.

One way to focus on truth is to concentrate on God's Word (perhaps a favorite passage), His blessings for you, His will for you, or His mission for you. Or, focus on who God says you are. The promises of God would also be a powerful image for this focal point. Other great images to consider are visuals of Jesus conquering death and fighting off the forces of darkness.

What does "true" mean to you when it comes to God?

WHATEVER IS NOBLE

> *But God demonstrates His own love for us in this: While we were still sinners, Christ died for us.* (Romans 5:8)

A noble person is someone who does good for others when they do not have to. They are a person of high moral character, and they are willing to lower themselves for another.

For you, this picture might be of a family member or someone else in your life who chose to help you out when they didn't have to, and their action changed everything for the better.

Jesus's majesty and nobility are clear in His death on the cross and in the way the Spirit takes care of us every single day, tending to our needs. God's patience and compassion are noble, too. Satan wants our shame to keep us stuck in feelings of worthlessness, convincing us that we will never live up to God's best. But God forgives, and He makes people and things new.

Noble thoughts should help you to feel love and acceptance. They should help you see your value as someone who is a beloved child of God.

What does noble mean to you when it comes to God?

WHATEVER IS RIGHT

It is right for me to feel this way about all of you, since I have you in my heart...all of you share in God's grace with me.
(Philippians 1:7)

Our feelings and thoughts are not always right, so when we focus on rightness, we are exchanging wrong feelings and thoughts for ones that are aligned with God's thoughts and ways. Another way of looking at this is to think about things that are good. The goodness or rightness you think about can be in relation to situations or relationships.

For many years, I (Ronnie) had an anger problem. During my residency, I'd feel it come on. I'd get frustrated, and my lower back would start to get a burning sensation. Before I knew it, my frustration had multiplied due to the chaos around and within me, and the burning in my back had traveled all the way up my spine. By that point, I'd be losing my temper more often than not. I knew I needed a solution.

For a while, I tried telling myself not to be angry. That didn't work at all.

Then I tried getting my mind off what was making me mad by listing all the books of the Bible, which I had learned to do when I was ten. I had to concentrate when I got to all those minor prophets, and I had to let go of the things that were upsetting me in order to get the names right: Hosea, Joel, Amos, Obadiah, Jonah, Micah, Nahum, Habakkuk, Zephaniah, Haggai, Zechariah, and Malachi. I didn't realize it at the time, but this practice was allowing me to take two steps back and think about what I needed to do instead of what I was feeling. I was able to calm down and ask God for His fruit of the Spirit to take over.

When using the algorithm, it's important to think about what is right and good for the situation and for those around us. When we let our anxiety, fear, or other negative emotions affect our relationships, we are losing the battle. We must aim for rightness. I knew that being easily angered in my residency was not of God and that I had to change. I needed to have a posture of love, joy, peace, patience, kindness, goodness, gentleness, faithfulness, and self-control. Once I identified the *right* thinking, I was able to identify thoughts that would put me in the right headspace and quiet my frustration.

Becoming anxious or stressed over circumstances will negatively affect our relationship with God. We can't control other people, but we can control the way that we respond. When we are in right relationship with God, we trust Him and rely on Him to handle the things that get to us. If we abide in Him, He will come through. My (Ronnie's) self-control is much better because God has produced good fruit in me as I yield it to Him. I went from having to intentionally calm myself to having calmness be reflexive in me. That's the way God's process works. With practice, we are shaped into who He has called us to be.

What does right mean to you when it comes to God?

WHATEVER IS PURE

Whoever dwells in the shelter of the Most High will rest in the shadow of the Almighty. I will say to the LORD, "He is my refuge and my fortress, my God, in whom I trust." (Psalm 91:1–2)

In her book *The Christian's Secret of a Happy Life*, Hannah Whitall Smith writes about how she heard a woman talk about things that happen in the life of a Christian that don't look like they come from the hand of God, such as illness, loss, defeat, abuse, and suffering—whatever it may be that takes away from our joy and from experiencing the presence of God. She said God had shown her that His presence protects us and that He is still in control despite the difficulties and trials we go through, working in them to fulfill His eternal purposes. We will experience hurt and suffering and pain, but when we rest in the Spirit of a loving Father, we will experience these things in a much different way than if we were to have no hope at all in the Lord. There will be evil in the world, but we have access to God's protection, peace, and wholeness. Bad things might happen to us, but they do not have to define or change us.

I (Ronnie) have found that my Christian walk is most impactful to others when I've gone through some really tough, bad things. When people have seen me maintain my Christian hope amid such struggles, that's when they've been most drawn to my Savior. That's when they've started to ask questions about my faith.

Our Savior had to suffer. He was not immune to the evil and bad in this world, but He did show us how to rely on the Holy Spirit and on our walk with God to shield us from allowing those things to affect the work that He is doing within us. If we follow Jesus, we will have to pick up our own crosses and accept that there will be struggle, there will be hardship. But there will also be hope, and that is what purity is all about.

I (Ronnie) envision the Holy Spirit wrapped around me like filter paper. He filters out of my life all the evil in this world except for that which God can "work together for the good." (See Romans 8:28.) How comforting it is to know that our loving Father will only allow those things in our life that have the potential to make us more like Jesus.

As a people living with the hope found in Christ, we should be able to look for the pure things in life, for the hand of God that is present even in suffering and evil. Titus 1:15 says, *"To the pure, all things are pure."* Do you live in accordance with this truth? Do you believe it? When you're facing down your most anxious thoughts, are you able to allow the Spirit to show you something pure and holy in the midst of that struggle? How has He protected you in the midst of suffering in the past? How has He walked you through pain and difficulty?

What does pure mean to you when it comes to God?

WHATEVER IS LOVELY

> *One thing I ask from the LORD, this only do I seek: that I may dwell in the house of the LORD all the days of my life, to gaze on the beauty of the LORD and to seek him in his temple.*
>
> (Psalm 27:4)

There are so many lovely things all around us, but what encapsulates the word *lovely* to you? What fully embodies exquisite beauty? For me (Ronnie), when I think of something lovely, I think of heaven.

We can let our imaginations run wild when it comes to what heaven will look like and be like, and it still won't come close to reality. Heaven will be everything that we wish for and more, and the loveliest thing in heaven will be God Himself. He will radiate beauty, and that beauty will fall on everything around Him. He will reign completely and fully, and everything broken will be made right.

When I think of the loveliness of heaven, I think of walking the streets of gold and of being in the presence of God in the cool of the day, just as Adam and Eve had the opportunity to do. And God will take the beauty of heaven and bring it down here on earth. He will make this world a beautiful, wonderful place in which to live. Everything will be complete and as it should be.

This is what "lovely" means to me, but what does it mean to you? What is incredibly beautiful to you? A child's laugh? A rushing river? A lifelong friendship? A restored relationship? When you think of the most beautiful thing, what comes to mind?

What does lovely mean to you when it comes to God?

WHATEVER IS ADMIRABLE

> *Let us then approach God's throne of grace with confidence, so that we may receive mercy and find grace to help us in our time of need.* (Hebrews 4:16)

Who or what is most deserving of respect? Is there a mentor, a coach, a friend, or a family member in your life who has obtained your ultimate respect and admiration? Perhaps, when you think of something admirable, you imagine a situation that someone handled very well or a difficult decision that someone navigated with selflessness and respect.

For me (Ronnie), when it comes to what is admirable, I think of God on His throne. No other image comes nearly as close to grabbing my attention and bringing up within me feelings of respect. I think of God sitting with His arms open wide, ready to give me a hug. I hear Him say to me, "Ronnie, come on up here, and let's talk about all that stuff that is upsetting you. I've got this. I am here to make all things new. Rest here in My lap." And that, to me, is more than worthy of my admiration because it shows His mercy and grace, both of which I so desperately need. I don't deserve any of what He gives me, but He makes it possible for me to step into His kingdom. Is there anything more admirable than that?

What does admirable mean to you when it comes to God?

WHATEVER IS EXCELLENT OR PRAISEWORTHY

> Lord, our Lord, how majestic is your name in all the earth! You have set your glory in the heavens. (Psalm 8:1)

Excellence is rooted in perfection, and something that is perfect (or above reproach) is worthy of praise. Of course the only perfect person or thing in this universe is God our King, so this focal point should chiefly draw your attention to the Lord.

When you think of an aspect of God that is excellent or praiseworthy, you might think of His mercy, His compassion, His creativity, or His justice. You might think of the ways He has moved in your life or the miracles He has done. For me (Ronnie), I think of how He has allowed me to become part of His family. I see myself as a child of the King, and, through that, I am able to look past the darkness and despair of this world to see the bigger picture. Too often, I place all of my hope in this world, but it only lets me down. I try to control things here, and that's when I get anxious. That's when I get stressed and fearful, because the reality is that I have *no* control!

Yet, when I focus on God and His kingdom, I'm able to accept this life for what it is, knowing that there is a greater calling, a greater purpose, and a greater place for me. And the best part is that I don't have to control a thing. I don't have to stress or worry. God is doing the work, and that is both excellent and praiseworthy.

What does excellent and praiseworthy mean to you when it comes to God?

In chapter 14, we will explore how this all comes together to create new pathways in our thinking.

14

CREATING NEW PATHWAYS

We've explored the focal points of Philippians 4:8—whatever is true, noble, right, pure, lovely, admirable, excellent, and praiseworthy—and we've seen how to personalize these concepts. Now we have to practice thinking about them. This is what brings the greatest impact. We have to sear these images and truths into our brains, creating new pathways so that, when we feel anxious or stressed or hopeless, we are able to stop those negative thoughts in their tracks and think about positive images and truths instead.

This requires "taking every thought captive" (see 2 Corinthians 10:5)—even the negative thoughts that you are convinced are protecting you from disaster. It requires *thinking* instead of *feeling* your way through your anxiety. It requires running every thought through the test of asking yourself, "Is this true? Is this noble? Is this right? Is this pure, lovely, admirable, excellent, or praiseworthy?"

I (Ronnie) found it helpful to write down my personalized algorithm and keep it in my pocket. When situations, thoughts, or anything else would attack my peace, I would pull it out and read it. Out loud, if possible. Believe it or not, the bathroom was a very spiritual place for me. Whenever I was stressed, I would go in there, pull out my paper, and read my algorithm. The people at work probably thought I drank way too much water!

At first, it might be difficult for you to do this on your own. Your anxious thoughts might be so strong and prevalent that you have a hard time seeing through their lies. This is when community comes to the rescue. Going to a trusted friend and asking them for their perspective on the thoughts you are having can help you see things more clearly. It also will invite that person into your struggle, and they may become an important support or part of your journey.

The Bible tells us that Paul was mentored by Barnabas, and then Paul went on to mentor Timothy. This shows the power and beauty of community, of iron sharpening iron. (See Proverbs 27:17.) Each of us needs someone we can go to in times of struggle and confusion. As we learn and grow, we can then be the iron sharpening the next group of believers.

All of this is to help us move toward reflexiveness, to a place where we have *"set [our] minds on things above, not on earthly things"* (Colossians 3:2). As mentioned previously, reflexiveness does not come naturally to us. The Christian life is not automatic. Just because we believe and follow Jesus doesn't mean that we know all the Scriptures, have all the answers, and behave the way we should 100 hundred percent of the time. Not only is that impossible, but it's not what God had in mind! We are living, breathing beings who are formed in Christ over time as we rely on the Spirit within us and the community of believers around us. But, more than that, we can continually have an awareness of the "manifest presence of God."

I (Ronnie) first read about this concept of the "manifest presence" in the book *Healing Prayer* by David Chotka and Maxie Dunnam, who write, "The term 'Manifest Presence' is a classic theological term. It refers to a tangible sense of God's power becoming evident to human senses."[30] Most of us have experienced this tangible sense at

---

30. David Chotka and Maxie Dunnam, *Healing Prayer* (New Kensington, PA: Whitaker House, 2023), 18n2.

least once in our lives. Such an experience is more than knowing that the Spirit is within you or sensing a voice of assurance or guidance in your head or a conviction in your heart. The manifest presence is the awesome power of God around you and before you in a way that you can almost feel on your skin. It's that sense you get when you're in a very difficult situation, and yet you feel peace. I've experienced God's manifest presence when I've had to tell parents that their child is no longer with us. In those heartbreaking times, I would pray hard and ask the Lord to help and lead me, and He would show up. He'd give me strength for that moment and comfort and empathy for the parents. I have watched time and again as God took what would have been a very difficult conversation and used it for His glory. Living with the manifest presence of God will change your life, and the algorithm is just one of the many paths you can take to welcome more of that powerful presence. God longs to walk with all His children like He walked with Adam and Eve. He longs to be *with us*, not just in us.

IDENTIFYING YOUR TRIGGERS

The algorithm is therefore designed so that the moment you are triggered by a situation or an anxious or fearful or ugly thought, you identify the emotion you are feeling (essentially saying the name of the thing or the feeling or the memory that is causing you to go down a dark path) and replace it with thoughts that are true, noble, right, pure, lovely, admirable, excellent, and praiseworthy—thoughts that invite the presence of God. The process goes like this:

1. Something bad happens (or you suddenly have an anxious or fearful thought).
2. You have an initial reaction (fear, questioning God, feeling sorry for yourself, or another response).
3. You make a decision to accept where you are emotionally and respond to your reaction by drawing toward God using the algorithm.

The more you do this, the more you will reshape your brain and the way that you see and interact with the world around you, forever changing your life by making room for the presence of God. This is how you *mentally* take two steps back and gain control *emotionally* and *spiritually*.

Let's review the above three steps by looking at a specific example:

1. You receive bad news about your health.
2. Your initial reaction is one of fear, worry, and anger. You can't believe that God would allow this to happen to you, and all you can think about is the long road ahead and the pain and suffering this will cause you and your loved ones.
3. Then, you decide to invite God into your journey by replacing those thoughts with thoughts of Him, His goodness, and His majesty. You still feel a bit scared and upset by the news, but you also feel peace, knowing that God is with you, and this peace begins to transform your perspective.

Of course, a bad health diagnosis is one of the hardest things we can navigate, so let's look at another example of what this process might look like for a less significant trigger:

1. You are running late for work, and the traffic on your commute is at a standstill.
2. Your initial reaction is panic. You are mad at yourself for not having left home earlier, and you begin to anticipate your boss's disappointed look and the stern, corrective email you will receive shortly after arriving at work. Your entire outlook for the day is crashing fast.
3. You decide to take two steps back, realizing that you are doing your best as an employee and that the traffic situation is completely outside your control. You begin replacing your self-criticizing thoughts with the presence of God by focusing on His love and faithfulness. Before you know it, you start to think about all the good that you bring to

your job, and you decide that your boss's reaction won't dictate the joy and peace that you have for that day.

By tracking your triggers and responses, you will be able to reveal thought patterns and behaviors that are contributing to your triggers. You might find that you always cower when thinking about your boss's potential lack of approval, or that you struggle to maintain your sense of worth when you aren't picture-perfect. Knowing the things, people, or situations that cause you to emotionally spiral is crucial to creating new patterns and behaviors that will invite the presence of God and bring mental health. (We will talk more about this in the next chapter.)

BUILD YOUR ALGORITHM

Your algorithm should be tailored to fit your needs, your triggers, and the way you worship God. Let's build an algorithm together, using various ideas presented earlier, so that you can get a better sense of what it could entail and how it could be used in your particular situation.

What is true?

- What lies does Satan tend to tell you? Which of these have you accepted, and why?
- What truths (from the Bible, your situation, and the people involved) might help you dispel those lies?

What is noble?

- What does it mean to be noble? What does that look like *to you*?
- What is the most noble act you can think of?
- What do you think would be a noble response in this circumstance?

What is right?

- What is the right thing to do in this situation?

- How might your family need to see you trusting God in this circumstance?

What is pure?

- What is something that is unblemished? A child's laugh? A flower?
- What does God's pure provision look like?
- What do you think "God's best" would be in this situation? And how might He surprise you with something even better?

What is lovely?

- When you think of a lovely experience, who is there with you? Or are you by yourself? What are you doing? What makes it lovely?
- How could the presence of God be lovely in your life right now?

What is admirable?

- When was a time you acted admirably?
- When did someone do something admirable for you? How did you feel? What did you experience?
- What could be admirable in this situation?

What is excellent?

- Think about human excellence compared with God's excellence.
- How have you seen God's perfection and excellence in your life?
- How can you trust God's excellence to work in your current situation?

What is praiseworthy?

- What has God done in your life or the life of someone else that deserves praise?

- How might He move in your life and bring change in a way that stirs up even more praise within you?

Take some time to think through each of these questions as you build your algorithm. Consider your unique story, your faith journey, and the way that you connect with and worship God. The result, based on the above questions and those from the previous chapter, should be the beginnings of an algorithm that is entirely unique to you and full of potential for God's presence in your life.

Think of your algorithm as a work in progress. You will likely adjust it over time as you find what works for you and what doesn't. But, more important, the more God moves, the more memories and experiences you will have to draw upon. And that is the beauty of having God in your life. He is active and working, and, every day, He gives you something new for which to praise Him.

◇ ◇ ◇

WELLNESS EXERCISE: A DAILY QUIET TIME

Some time ago, I (Ronnie) was working on fixing a dirt path that runs through the family property. It was eroding to the point where it was becoming unusable, and I needed to correct that. I bought some sod and worked to build it back up. Around noon, I decided to take a lunch break, so I went back home. Then, a thunderstorm hit, but by early afternoon, the storm had gone and the skies were once again clear, so I returned to work on the path. The only problem was that all my hard work had been undone. One storm had removed all the progress I had made.

Our emotions and triggers can be like that thunderstorm. They can come in fast, and, in a matter of moments, all of our hard work can be wiped out. That's why preparation is mandatory. It's not just a matter of knowing your algorithm. It's a matter of changing your lifestyle to be in line with the promises of God, because God will always show up. No matter what, He's going to be there. But His movement in our lives is often dependent on whether or not we are prepared and putting in the effort. And one of the simplest ways to do that is to have a daily quiet time in which you pray and read the Bible. It doesn't have to be sixty minutes or even thirty minutes long. You can start by spending five minutes before the Lord where you get quiet and come into His presence. Then, you can run through a checklist similar to this:

- What's on your mind? What is the state of your emotions?
- Present your concerns to God in an honest way.
- Read a passage from the Bible; length is not important—truth is.
- Sit in God's presence until you feel you are ready to start your day (or to conclude your session if you do this at another time during the day, or to end your day if you do this at bedtime).
- Check in with God throughout the day, especially if you begin to feel anxious or fearful.

That's it. Just spend five minutes (or more), and you can set yourself up for success when you need to implement the algorithm.

15

MAPPING THE JOURNEY

If our goal is to abide in Christ and be in the presence of the God of peace, and if thinking about the focal points in Philippians 4 helps us to get to that place of peace (or at the very least *closer* to it), then it follows that this algorithm or this process by which we experience transformation should not be taken lightly. To get the most out of the transformation process, we should pay attention to what happens each and every time we feel fear or anxiety and engage with Philippians 4.

To help us do this, we use a simple worksheet called the "Anxiety Algorithm Thought Record."[31] This Thought Record (see pages 145–149) will allow you to track what happens whenever you experience a trigger and engage the algorithm seeking peace and health.

The worksheet provides a ten-step flow so that you can record what happens from the moment a triggering event starts through the process of engaging the algorithm and identifying the outcome. Prompts at the bottom of each column or step are there to help you

---

31. The Anxiety Algorithm Thought Record is adapted from Carol Vivyan's "Thought Record Sheet—7 Column" (2010) available on http://getselfhelp.co.uk/ and adapted from Padesky (1995). Used by permission.

provide the best insight, and the blank space is there for you to write down what you experienced, what happened, and so on. A good time to complete this worksheet is before bed as you reflect on your day. What brought on fear or anxiety? What put you on edge? Start with those broad questions and then record your experiences in a notebook, working through the Thought Record as you do so.

By keeping a record of your algorithm process, you should be able to identify anxiety patterns, correct those patterns, and track your overall progress. If you find yourself implementing the algorithm without much success, the Thought Record should provide some insight as to why. If you experience a great breakthrough in using the algorithm, the Thought Record should be able to help you identify what led up to that, and so on.

Let's walk through the worksheet together.

STEP 1: WHAT HAPPENED? (SITUATION/TRIGGER)

It can be hard to know exactly what sets you off in a given moment. You may think that your anxiety was triggered by traffic or parenting or a rough meeting at work when, in reality, its roots go much deeper. While you don't have to pinpoint the cause of each episode perfectly, it's important to try—even if you're unsure or just guessing. The process of asking yourself what happened, who were you with, how you reacted, and why is important, whether you have it all figured out or not. Simply engaging this process of asking questions will, in time, sharpen your awareness of yourself and your triggers. The more you can get in touch with your emotions and understand why you feel the way you feel, the more aware you will be.

When you address this step, feel free to indicate your confidence level. If you're certain that you've identified the trigger, say so. If you're unsure, that's okay, too, and you can indicate that. Recording your certainty level will help you when you come back to review your Thought Records.

You will also want to identify if the trigger itself was the problem, or if the trigger made you think of a different situation, causing a reaction. For example, someone with PTSD is often triggered by an event that has nothing to do with their actual trauma, anxiety, and fear. They may be in their home on the Fourth of July, and the sound of celebratory fireworks reminds them of the battlefield, triggering an episode. The fireworks were the triggers, yes, but they were not the root of the problem.

This type of reaction can happen not only to veterans but also to victims of sexual abuse, physical abuse, bullying, and health issues. So, be aware: the thing that triggers you might not be the core problem. For example, you may be walking through a store, and your brain sees someone whose likeness triggers memories of someone who abused you in the past. It may take serious consideration and practice to understand your triggers.

I (James) worked with a woman who was suddenly stricken with terrible anxiety when she became a grandmother. It took time, but we were able to uncover that she was abused by a relative. It was the birth of her grandchild and her unconscious fears that something similar would happen to the child that triggered her PTSD symptoms.

For many of us, however, our triggers are less traumatic. I (James) remember when I was visiting my parents, and I had my boys with me. When we went to leave, my mom watched as my boys piled into the car. She turned to me and said, "Don't forget to buckle them up."

I was thirty-five years old. I didn't have a history of accidents, and, on top of that, I was studying to be a psychologist! I knew the importance of car seats and buckling up. I had to realize that my mother's comment wasn't about me. She was triggered by fear, by the thought of something happening to her grandchildren. She wasn't their mother, and she wasn't going to be in the car with us, so she was responding in the only way she knew how: she was telling me what to do in an attempt to ensure our safety. It was the only thing she could think of to get some control over the situation.

Her trigger was our getting into the car. Her brain began to imagine all the bad things that could happen—the "what-if's"—and then the worry hit.

Those are examples of triggers that call back to previous trauma or anxiety versus triggers that are more in-the-moment.

STEP 2: HOW DO I FEEL (FROM 0–100 PERCENT)?/ BODY SENSATIONS

In this step, you're going to focus on how you feel physically and emotionally. You'll identify single words, such as *afraid, embarrassed, sad, alone, angry*, and so on. If you have trouble coming up with words that accurately describe exactly how you feel, you can find many "emotion wheels" online that provide a way to pinpoint a specific emotion. For example, you may know that you feel sad, but that term may seem too vague to you. Having a list of more precise synonyms can help you uncover additional emotions that are similar to "sad" but more specific. You may realize that you're actually feeling discouraged, depressed, and/or hurt. Words like these are much more descriptive and helpful when dealing with an anxiety episode.

The body can also respond when you have an emotional reaction. You can record any physical changes you sense in your body. You may, for example, feel a pit in your stomach. You may feel parts of your body start to sweat. You may feel a burning sensation in your lower back (just as I [Ronnie] talked about earlier when I would become angry). Knowing what happens in your body can help you quickly identify when you are having an emotional response and, possibly, what emotion you are experiencing. I (James) know that when my earlobes feel like they are getting hot, I am either anxious or angry. I typically notice my earlobes before I realize the emotion itself.

Once you have your word or words, give each of them a percentage rating. Of all of the things you are feeling, you might be 20 percent sad, 40 percent lonely, 25 percent stressed. This is an important way to get to know your body and to anticipate what you're feeling.

Emotions happen; we were created with the capacity for emotion, but sometimes we feel emotion without fully recognizing it. Identifying what you felt leading up to your anxiety or panic will help you to get ahead of the curve. If you know that you tend to feel very overlooked and hopeless before you begin to experience deep depression, then you can be on alert for those feelings and do what needs to be done to get help before the depression settles in.

This exercise isn't just for those who struggle with serious trauma and debilitating depression. It's also for those who are sometimes anxious or stressed. We can learn to recognize the warning signs that indicate an episode of anxiety or stress is around the corner, and, once we know the warning signs, we can pay attention to how our bodies respond. In that moment when my mother told me to buckle up my kids, I felt discouraged. I've found that, when I'm discouraged, I slouch. This was something that I'd done for years but wasn't aware of until I began to record my thoughts and anxious episodes so that I could understand myself better and benefit fully from God's peace. You might have other physical triggers. Stomach issues, sweating, shaking, tightness in the chest—these and more can all indicate anxiety, stress, or fear.

STEP 3: WHAT THOUGHTS WERE TROUBLESOME? (UNHELPFUL/UNTRUE THOUGHTS OR IMAGES)

Often, when we have an unhelpful thought, it is also one that is irrational. It causes worry about something that is completely outside our control. For example, you might have a fear of flying. But it's a very different thing to be merely afraid of the possibility of crashing versus being afraid of a crash because, while you are on a flight, you see that one of the airplane's exit doors is not properly secured. One of those thoughts is irrational and unhelpful—the other may be life-saving.

In order to determine if your thoughts are unhelpful/untrue, take two steps back. Inhale deeply, hold that breath, and then exhale. Begin to think about your Philippians 4 focal areas. Then, think specifically about what exactly it is you are afraid of and what your brain is telling you about that thing. For example, you may have been triggered by someone telling you that they want to go on a vacation with you, but the thing you're actually afraid of is the plane flight. Take time to imagine that scenario, thinking in images as well as with words. Then, ask yourself the following questions:

- What button is this pressing for me?
- What is the worst thing that could happen here?
- Is that fear rooted in reality, or is it a "what if"?

Anxiety preys upon thoughts that are irrational, thoughts that are formed upon a fear of what could be rather than what is. Anxiety takes those thoughts and convinces you that not only are they *possible*, but they are also *probable*. When I was getting ready to drive home with my sons after visiting with my parents, my mother feared for our safety because her thoughts told her that we were destined to get into a car accident. While that danger must have felt very present and real to her, the likelihood of it happening was very slim. It was a "what if" thought that spiraled out of control and took my mother captive.

These "what ifs" cause worry and fear because the more we ruminate on and entertain them, the more they take root. This is how people end up never leaving their house or refusing to get on an airplane. They become so overtaken by their fear of the unknown that they stop living their lives.

The unhelpful and untrue thoughts you harbor might not make a lot of sense to others, but that doesn't matter. They make sense to you, and so you need to be the one to unravel them—to get to the root of what is going on by taking two steps back and trying to see them clearly.

When we take hold of such thoughts and begin to see them for what they are (rather than what they seem to be), we can begin to replace them with new thoughts. You may have grown up with an anxious parent who told you repeatedly to stay safe, to get off the playground, to *not* jump and leap and climb like the other kids. Eventually, you began to believe that you shouldn't do those things because you're incapable of doing so without getting hurt. This negative self-belief may have wreaked havoc when you grew older and needed to take a "leap of faith" to apply for a new job or start a new relationship, but all you heard was your anxious parent's voice, and so you didn't move forward with your life.

This is why identifying unhelpful and untrue thoughts is so important: it will give you the opportunity to replace those negative thoughts with good, uplifting, positive ones. We will talk more about this later.

STEP 4: WHAT IS TRUE ABOUT THOSE THOUGHTS? (FACTS THAT *SUPPORT* THE UNHELPFUL/UNTRUE THOUGHTS)

Now it's time to put those thoughts on trial. Ask yourself:

- What is absolutely true about my worst-case scenario?
- When it comes to this situation, which of my fears are valid and legitimate?

In the scenario with the seat belts, my mother might have said something like, "It's rush hour, and more accidents happen during rush hour, so there is a possibility that something bad could happen."

Someone afraid of flying might say, "I don't know the pilot, so I don't know if I can trust them, and the weather is looking bad today. So, I do know for a fact that conditions will be more difficult."

Whatever it may be, state firmly and plainly the truth about your fears. You need to recognize their validity before you can see them as anything else than a threat.

STEP 5: WHAT AM I FAILING TO SEE? (FACTS THAT PROVIDE EVIDENCE *AGAINST* THE UNTRUE OR UNHELPFUL THOUGHT)

You've identified your valid concerns, so now it's time to uncover the evidence that reveals any false thoughts that you might have. Ask yourself:

- Am I reacting to an opinion or a feeling instead of a fact? (Let's return to the airplane example. Having a fear of flying without knowing that there is anything wrong with the plane or with the pilot—even though you don't know the pilot personally—is a fear that is rooted in emotion and opinion, not fact.)
- Do I trust the people involved? (This would have been an important question for my mother to ask herself when she advised us about wearing seat belts. Of course, she trusted me! Reminding herself of that would have helped to alleviate her fear that day.)
- What have others said about this? How do my trusted friends approach the same topic?

This part of the process is all about parsing out what is legitimate fear and what is anxiety, worry, or stress based on past trauma or out-of-control what-if scenarios. It will not entirely erase the possibility that your worst fear could be actualized—at the end of the day, we can't know for sure that the plane won't crash. But it can help you to reframe your mindset so that the algorithm is more effective, which leads us to step 6.

STEP 6: USE THE ALGORITHM

Up to this point, we've been rooting ourselves in physical, mental, and emotional realities, but it's time to invite Jesus into our fears and concerns. It's time to really pursue Him and engage with the Spirit, and one of the easiest ways to jump-start this is to take two steps back (if you haven't done so already). Take a breath. Calm yourself.

Quiet the things in your mind that are demanding your attention, and then run through your algorithm, reshaping your thoughts to reflect things that are true, noble, right, pure, lovely, admirable, excellent, and praiseworthy. Spend time with each of those focal points. Then, ask yourself:

- In this situation, what do I have control over?

Say whatever comes to mind! It may seem silly. You may respond with a firm, "Nothing!" or something specific, such as, "I can plan my day to reduce the likelihood that X might happen."

It's important, though, to recognize the things you don't have control over. Even by telling me to buckle up my kids, my mother still had no control over whether or not they would be hurt in an accident. Acknowledging our own inability to control a situation might seem defeating, but it's actually an important step toward being able to let go and turn our back on what is making us panic or worry. By recognizing that you don't have control over your situation, you can give it to God and tell your brain and body to stop wasting so much energy on it.

STEP 7: CLAIM THE PROMISES OF GOD

The promises of God are incredibly powerful. There is nothing in the world that is fully, completely true except for God and what He has promised us. While doubt will always creep into our minds, the beauty of God's promises is that they are true whether we can fully receive them or not.

There is a story in the ninth chapter of Mark that has been a significant help to my (Ronnie's) doubt. A father brings his son to Jesus and asks that, if it is possible, would He please heal his son. Jesus replies that all things are possible to those who believe. The father makes a wonderful confession that has been so relevant in my life and in the lives of numerous people with whom I have shared this story. He says, *"I do believe; help me overcome my unbelief!"* (Mark 9:24). How reassuring it has been to me and so many others that Jesus does not require perfect faith with no doubt for His promises to be true. Really, all He requires is that we come to Him with anything in our lives that is a problem. He can do the rest. So, even though doubt will always threaten to get in the way of our going to God to claim His promises, it does not need to stop us from praying those promises, and it does not stop Him from moving. Anywhere that Scripture says God will do something for us or that He has done something, that is a promise.

Begin by asking this question:

- What does Scripture tell me about this situation and/or about God's love for me and His character?

Dig into that. Really think about how the reality of a Most High God who loves you changes your situation today.

Some verses that are helpful in this process are:

God has said, "Never will I leave you; never will I forsake you". So we say with confidence, "The Lord is my helper; I will not be afraid. What can mere mortals do to me?" (Hebrews 13:5–6)

Trust in the LORD with all your heart and lean not on your own understanding; in all your ways submit to him, and he will make your paths straight. (Proverbs 3:5–6)

Now to him who is able to do immeasurably more than all we ask or imagine, according to his power that is at work within us, to him be glory in the church and in Christ Jesus throughout all generations, for ever and ever! Amen. (Ephesians 3:20–21)

Who shall separate us from the love of Christ? Shall trouble or hardship or persecution or famine or nakedness or danger or sword? As it is written: "For your sake we face death all day long; we are considered as sheep to be slaughtered." No, in all these things we are more than conquerors through him who loved us. (Romans 8:35–37)

Come to me, all you who are weary and burdened, and I will give you rest. (Matthew 11:28)

Whatever you have learned or received or heard from me, or seen in me—put it into practice. And the God of peace will be with you. (Philippians 4:9)

Claim these promises with conviction. Despite your doubt, despite your fear, state the promises of God with the belief that He can and will deliver you. Over time, this practice will create a new way of thinking within you, a new way for your brain to process and handle stress and anxiety.

What promise of God do you need to claim for hope, reassurance, or encouragement? Write it down and bring it to God in prayer. The more you do this, the more reflexive it will become for you to seek His presence when you face anxiety or stress. After practicing this for some months, I (Ronnie) found myself automatically claiming the promises of God every time anxiety or fear began to well up within me. Those truths allowed me to stop my destructive thoughts before they got hold of me. And now, years into my practicing the algorithm, I'm such a freer, more joyful, more positive person. Relying on God's promises has completely changed my life.

STEP 8: FIND A DIFFERENT PERSPECTIVE

With this step, you try to replace your existing thoughts and images with ones that are true, helpful, and possibly life-changing. In doing so, you can find a different perspective—an alternative, more realistic, and biblical perspective. Here are some questions to get you there:

- Is there another way of seeing this situation? Is there a bigger picture that I'm missing?
- How might a godly friend view the same situation? What would they say about it?

- Is this fear or situation as important as it seems? Or is my body reacting to something that is more of a "what-if" fear than an actual threat?

Returning once more to the example of my (James's) mom and the seat belts, she could have thought about my perspective—how these are my children, and I will do anything to protect them—and realized that I was going to buckle them in and drive as carefully as possible. Realizing these truths could have eased her fears about their getting hurt.

This step is all about moving away from worry over what is possible, and focusing more on what is probable, knowing that God is with us and watching over us. Will something painful or difficult or scary happen to you tomorrow? Maybe. Possibly. But it's not a for-sure thing. What *is* sure is that God loves you and is with you. Even if He doesn't take away the thing that grips you, He absolutely will make beauty from ashes.

STEP 9: PRAY TO THE HOLY SPIRIT

Take this newfound perspective and the promises of God, and bring them together in prayer to the Holy Spirit. Ask Him for specific help with your particular fears and concerns, using the worksheet to fuel your prayers. Tell Him exactly what is bothering you and why. Tell Him your fears, your insecurities. Tell Him exactly how much you are impacted by these things, and be honest about your desire for a breakthrough. State God's truths back to Him, be open about your faith or lack thereof, and give Him your doubt.

God delights in your vulnerability and honesty, and using the steps on this worksheet will help you enter into a conversation with Him in a posture of complete openness.

STEP 10: OUTCOME: RE-RATE YOUR FEELINGS (FROM 0-100%)

Write down what happened after you went through the nine previous steps, which incorporate the algorithm. Your description could be one word, a sentence, or a whole page of notes. It could be a drawing or a poem.

Maybe God really showed up and met you as you were doing the worksheet and spoke truth into you through the Holy Spirit. Maybe you went from feeling total anxiety to having a sense of peace and awe.

Maybe you didn't feel much of anything. Or maybe your fears subsided for a bit, but they didn't go away. Maybe you prayed but didn't feel God's presence. Maybe you did every step of the worksheet and came away wondering if it was worth your time. Still, write that down. Record it.

Then, rate how you're feeling. I (James) have found that I need to warn my patients when I ask them to start using the Anxiety Algorithm Thought Record that they may record feeling sad at the beginning of this process and sad at the end of it. That is why we ask them to use the percentages to say *how* sad they feel. It may be unrealistic to think that they will go from being sad to being happy. It is more realistic to think they may go from 50 percent sad to 10 percent sad, which is a significant improvement. If you've found that your rating hasn't gotten any better, or if it's still significant enough to impact your day, repeat the algorithm, inviting God to again open your heart and mind so that you can feel His presence and see what He sees regarding your situation or concern.

If, after going through the algorithm two or three times, you feel just as bad, if not worse, talk to a friend. Invite someone into this space with you, and then try again. There is something impactful about human companionship when it comes to our deepest fears and anxieties. But please don't stop using the algorithm. It may take time, yet doing this process, engaging your loving Father, and focusing on His truth in your life will bring about change over time.

BUILD YOUR ALTAR

In the Old Testament, there were special altars or memorials of remembrance that God instructed His people to create, or which people created on their own initiative, in order to remember what God had done for them. If He had moved in a great way or saved them from destruction or worked a miracle, they would construct an altar of rocks so that, every time they passed through the area, they could remember God's goodness and faithfulness. (See, for example, Joshua 4:1–8.)

When you write down God's movement in your life, it's as if you're constructing an altar as a way to remember what He has done. What you experience may not be the full outcome you hoped for, but even a small step in the right direction is worthy of praise because it's a step toward healing as your brain begins to rewire and build new pathways to wholeness.

WELLNESS EXERCISE: THE THOUGHT RECORD METHOD

One of the best things you can do to move toward wellness is to literally document your process of going through the steps in the Anxiety Algorithm Thought Record worksheet. On pages 145–149, we have included an example of what the form can look like. You can make a copy of these pages, use a computer program such as Excel to make your own form, or simply create a form in a notebook or a list on your phone or tablet. Use whichever method is easiest for you.

Again, the most important thing is that you document and write down your process of working through the steps. Here's why: as we expressed earlier, it is much easier to discover patterns of thinking when you document them. As a therapist, it made it much easier for me (James) to see the pattern(s) of anxiety someone was dealing with when they used the form a dozen or so times and wrote down their process. In fact, it was pretty easy to see the patterns. Sometimes several themes related to anxiety emerged. I can't tell you how helpful this was to me and, even more, to the person I was trying to help.

That brings me to another point: if you are using this Thought Record tool and making sure to write everything down, and you still cannot see the pattern(s) of anxiety or fear, show the record to someone you really trust (a godly person) and ask them if they see any patterns in what you have written. You would be amazed at what others may be able to see because they have an outside perspective.

The most important thing you can do with the information in chapter 15 is to put it into practice. I (James) have seen this method work wonders for people. God can use it to reveal how your anxious thoughts and feelings are unfounded or lies or just not rooted in biblical truth. At the end of the day, it is God's truth, through His Spirit, that sets us free.

ANXIETY ALGORITHM THOUGHT RECORD

Step 1	What happened? (Situation/ Trigger) Ex: What happened? With whom? What? When?	
Step 2	How do I feel (from 0–100%)?/ Body sensations Ex: What emotion did I feel at that time? Anything else? How intense was it? What did I notice happen in my body?	

ANXIETY ALGORITHM THOUGHT RECORD

Step 3	What thoughts were troublesome? (unhelpful/ untrue thoughts or images) Ex: [Take Two Steps Back and breathe.] What went through my mind? What "button" is this pressing for me? What would be the worst thing about that thought or idea, or that could happen?	
Step 4	What is true about those thoughts? (Facts that *support* the unhelpful/ untrue thoughts) Ex: What are the facts? What facts do I have that the unhelpful thought(s) is totally true?	

ANXIETY ALGORITHM THOUGHT RECORD

Step 5	What am I failing to see? (Facts that provide evidence *against* the untrue or unhelpful thought) Ex: What facts do I have that the unhelpful thought(s) is NOT totally true? Is it possible that this is opinion rather than fact? What have others said about this?	
Step 6	Use the algorithm (whatever is true, noble right, pure, lovely, admirable, excellent, praiseworthy) Ex: [Take Two Steps Back!] What do I have control over? (My response.) What is out of my control? [Close your eyes and go through your algorithm.]	

ANXIETY ALGORITHM THOUGHT RECORD

Step 7	Claim the promises of God. Ex: Sample promise: "I will never leave you or forsake you." What am I afraid of? What does Scripture tell me about this situation and/or God's love and character?	
Step 8	Find a different perspective (an alternate, more realistic, and biblical perspective). Ex: Is there another way of seeing this situation? What is the bigger picture? How would a godly friend see this situation? Is this really as important as it seems?	

ANXIETY ALGORITHM THOUGHT RECORD

Step 9	Pray to the Holy Spirit. Ask Him for help, and try to be specific. Ex: [You may need to do your breathing exercise here.] Focus on what God is telling you. Be still before the Lord as best you can.	
Step 10	Outcome: Re-rate your feelings (from 0–100%). Ex: What emotions do I feel? How does my body feel? [You may need to go back through one or more of the steps if you do not yet feel any better.]	

The Anxiety Algorithm Thought Record is adapted from Carol Vivyan's "Thought Record Sheet —7 Column" (2010) available on http://getselfhelp.co.uk/ and adapted from Padesky (1995). Used by permission.

Part Three

OVERCOMING ANXIETY THROUGH STRONG RELATIONSHIPS

16

BUILDING STRONG RELATIONSHIPS, PART 1

Now that we've walked through the algorithm and offered insights for how to make it personal, let's apply the algorithm to gain a holistic view (heart, soul, mind, strength) of wellness.

We developed the Anxiety Algorithm from Philippians 4:8–9, but the whole book of Philippians is rich in advice for practical living—and isn't that what we're here for? To learn how to navigate life with a practical head for the things that truly matter?

ABUNDANT LIFE

How can we have a life of joy? How can we see the hope we have even in the midst of difficulty? Philippians has answers to these questions and more. Paul wanted the believers in the church at Philippi to experience the abundant life that Jesus promised, a life lived above circumstances, conflict, and need. Throughout Philippians, he focuses on not just believing what Jesus said, but also *living* it. In other words, he essentially emphasizes how to create new pathways in the brain—pathways that can absolutely revolutionize one's life.

Therefore, over the next few chapters of this book, we'll journey through highlights from the book of Philippians. Philippians focuses on mindset, which can transform your ability to change and become who you're supposed to be in every aspect of your life. Something shifts when we approach our relationship with God through the lens of who we are *becoming* rather than who we *are*. As *The Living Bible* puts it in Romans 5:2, *"For because of our faith, he has brought us into this place of highest privilege where we now stand, and we confidently and joyfully look forward to actually becoming all that God has had in mind for us to be."*

In particular, Philippians offers us so much insight from which to build emotional health, relational health, and spiritual health. It naturally lends itself to issues of the heart and emotional wellness, and it's an incredible guidebook for anyone struggling with anxiety, fear, and stress. Philippians is known as a book about joy, and that is one of its primary themes, especially the joy of knowing Jesus. Yet almost half the verses in the book of Philippians deal with relationships. Is this a coincidence? Or is it that relationships are one of the major factors in living a joyful life?

It might seem odd to talk about relationships in a book about anxiety, but our relationships are one of the greatest sources of peace or anxiety in our lives. Being in a community—and conversely being *without* community—makes a great difference in how we feel and how we approach life. When we're fearful or sad or hurting, there is something incredibly comforting about being with others. But dealing with people can be stressful—even the people we love. So, let's look next at what relationship means from the perspective of using the algorithm as a tool.

RECEIVING GRACE TOGETHER

Philippians is a letter to a church that Paul loved because of how they had partnered with him for the sake of the gospel. Naturally, then, it's a very relationship-focused book, and the fourth chapter of the book is all about relationships.

Our wellness starts with relationship—our relationship with God, our family members, fellow members of our church, and the world around us. The beginning of the book of Philippians is clear about this:

> *In all my prayers for all of you,* **I always pray with joy because of your partnership in the gospel** *from the first day until now, being confident of this, that he who began a good work in you will carry it on to completion until the day of Christ Jesus.*
>
> (Philippians 1:4–6)

A common bond with a common goal gives uncommon joy. Life as a Christian in Philippi was not easy, but this church body had found joy and purpose as they worked together for the cause of Christ. We are better when we have a shared mission because working together and being together gives us emotional strength.

When we fail at something, when we don't feel good about ourselves, when we are ashamed, Satan wants us to step away from our relationships—instead of moving toward them. He wants us to seek to be by ourselves because he knows that if we are alone, we are much more susceptible to the lies he tells us. Haven't you found this to be true in your own anxiety journey? Isolation and retreat seem appealing, but community breaks through the lies we have been believing. Together, we share in God's grace, and we can better hear His Spirit. Jesus tells us the truth, which sets us free. In God's community, we have all we need.

This is the beauty of grace. We can receive so much more than we deserve. This is for all of us: it's for you in your anxiety and struggles, it's for your neighbor whom you don't always get along with, and it's for your boss who rubs you the wrong way. This is an important aspect because the way that you see and treat others significantly affects the way that you see and treat yourself. And your ability to gain freedom from your anxiety and stress is directly tied to your relationship with others.

If someone does something to frustrate you, your initial reaction is perhaps to call them out and to hit back at them with what you feel they deserve. But while this response may feel good in the moment, it will only pull you further from peace and joy and community. It's not the way of the algorithm, and it's in this kind of response that bitterness develops. It's been said that bitterness is like drinking a cup of poison and expecting it to kill somebody else. It doesn't help you at all; it only hurts you.

Amazingly enough, bitterness doesn't seem to have been an issue in the Philippian church. (Of course, there was still conflict at times, which we will talk about in chapter 18.) Overall, the believers there had nurtured a beautiful community because of how they partnered together. The way they built one another up, lovingly corrected one another, and sought Jesus together created a strong bond that drew each one of them closer to Christ.

How does that work? And is it really possible for us to experience it today?

We believe it is. Implementing the lessons about relationships that we can learn from the Philippians will absolutely impact your relationships with others, with God, and even with yourself, making way for a heart, mind, soul, and strength that abides in Christ and is rid of the anxiety that would take hold of you.

For the rest of this chapter, we will explore the first three of seven key lessons in relationships that we can glean from the Philippian church. Then, in chapter 17, we will look at lessons 4–7.

RELATIONSHIP LESSONS FROM PHILIPPIANS

Lesson 1: Relationships Bring Wellness

Take a moment to see yourself in this picture that we have of the church at Philippi. Does it line up with your life today? Are you deep in Christian community? Do you rely on your brothers and sisters in Christ to speak into your life, and vice versa? Do you receive the corporate grace that is offered, or do you tend to fall for the trap of isolation and aloneness?

Maybe you're easy to get along with—so easy that you don't have a clear place within the group because you're always putting others first in a way that ends up being self-destructive. If so, you need to be more assertive in the best way—the Jesus way—by recognizing your strengths and contributing them to the group.

Or maybe you're expecting your community to be your everything, even relying on them more than you rely on Jesus. You exist in community because you want people to pour into your life over and over. You view your needs as the most important, the most urgent, and you're disappointed when your expectations aren't met. If so, you need to learn humility by deepening your relationship with your Lord and learning His thoughts and ways.

Or, maybe you're quite opinionated. You have an idea of how you think the group should operate and how each person in the group should live life, but instead of using the group's collective wisdom to filter through these opinions (or criticisms) in love, you bulldoze your way through, making the group into what you want it to be, not what the Spirit wants it to be. If so, you need to learn how to follow others and work with them.

We're all on a continuum between unhealth and health. We all bring some baggage into our relationships, but the main goal is to allow community to change us, not the other way around. So, take a look at your relationships and consider how you operate in them:

- How are you in relationship with others?
- What role do you tend to play in a group? What are the pros and cons of this role? What are the opportunities and pitfalls?
- Which people do you struggle to get along with?
- Which people tend to struggle to get along with you?

After considering these questions, you should also keep in mind that, in Romans 12:18, Paul tells us, *"If it is possible, as far as it depends on you, live at peace with everyone."* Because of sin and the human condition, this isn't always possible in community (which is why Paul clarifies that we are to do this *"if it is possible"*!). That's why the "Two Steps Back" approach works so well for relationships. When things get hard, when personalities clash, it's good to take two steps back. Do we give up on the other person? Absolutely not. But instead of engaging in a disagreement or conflict that isn't going anywhere and that is dominated by emotion, we can take two steps back and pray through the algorithm.

It can be tempting to build a wall when we've stepped away from someone, but that's why we need to stay in tune with the Spirit and with the community around us. Stepping away from a relationship should not be with the goal of permanent estrangement. It should be for the goal of reconciliation.

It's also important to note here that some people have diagnosed (or even undiagnosed) personality disorders. These people tend to pull a group toward unhealth, and it can be exceptionally difficult to live in harmony with them when they are not pursuing their own wellness. These individuals feel almost impossible to work with. The lens through which they see the world is different from most, and different in a disordered way. Personality disorders are more nurture than nature, learned over time, typically from growing up in a dysfunctional environment. However, extensive psychotherapy can help people to foster self-awareness of disordered habits and move toward health. One of the most significant barriers that those with personality disorders face is the fact that they often do not see the disorder in their life.

Most of us, however, don't fall into the realm of a clinical personality disorder, and we have an opportunity here to think through who we are and how we relate to others, either positively or negatively. As you consider these things, you may want to ask somebody to help you identify some of the details mentioned above about how you generally operate in relationship with others. A friend (not your spouse) would be ideal.

I (Ronnie) have a group of guys around me who will tell me the truth even if it hurts my feelings. They have this freedom because I've asked them to be honest with me. There have been times when they've gently confronted me for stepping out of line. It's not fun when this happens! But it's crucial for my growth, for my wellness, and for our relationship with each other because, while I may need these men beside me today, tomorrow they may need me!

Who might such a friend (or friends) be in your life? Again, consider bringing them into your journey as you seek to grow in your relationships while using the algorithm.

Lesson 2: It's Not Your Job to Fix People

Philippians 1:6 reads, *"Being confident of this, that he who began a good work in you will carry it on to completion until the day of Christ Jesus."* When we're in community, it can be tempting to think that it's our job to fix others, to fix the church, to fix the world. But that is God's job. Our job is to be faithful to what God has for *us to do*.

My (Ronnie's) oldest daughter Emily struggled with this very idea in her second year of college. She called me one day because she'd had enough: there were people around her, friends in her community, who were messing up and making terrible decisions, and Emily was at a loss as to what to do about it. She had done everything she could to show them the right path, but it wasn't working. These people were on unhealthy trajectories, and their lifestyles would eventually catch up with them. I could sense the burden Emily felt for these dear friends whom she longed to see happy and thriving.

So, we talked about it. Week after week, we discussed the situation, and I could see that it was bringing her lower and lower. I could tell that she was becoming depressed because of what was going on with her friends and because of her own inability to coach them out of their destructive patterns.

Finally, I had an idea. I asked Emily to take a three-by-five index card and write this on it: "Let God be God, and let Emily be Emily, and don't get the two confused." Then I advised her to put it by the light switch in her dorm room so that she would see it every time she left her room.

There are situations in which we have direct roles to play, and then there are situations in which the best thing for us to do is to hand everything over to God. It's our job to allow the Spirit to produce fruit within us and to let the world around us see that fruit. It's not our job to fix the world.

Emily could and should let her friends see her fruit, but it was not her job to inspect their fruit—not in a situation in which she wasn't directly spiritually responsible for their actions. If she were their parent, if they were employees of her ministry, or if she and they were in true accountability with one another, then she would have reason to dig in and inspect things further. But it was not her responsibility to make sure that all her friends' fruit was up to par.

This is a message that is especially important in marriage. Many times, wives tell their husbands regarding a problem they are dealing with, "I don't need you to fix it. I just need you to listen to me!"

How much of our anxiety, frustrations, and relational issues is caused by our trying to do God's job? God has pretty big shoes to fill, and it will wear us out trying to do His job! If we could just let go and stop trying to do God's job for Him, our anxiety might improve significantly.

Lesson 3: Pray Top-Down

Paul's prayer for the Philippians' discernment, priorities, and fruit is a powerful one:

> *And this is my prayer: that your love may abound more and more in knowledge and depth of insight, so that you may be able to discern what is best and may be pure and blameless for the day of Christ, filled with the fruit of righteousness that comes through Jesus Christ—to the glory and praise of God.*
>
> (Philippians 1:9–11)

The core message here is that when you love someone or something, you want to know as much about them as you can. If we approached God in the same way, He would reward us! He would give us knowledge and depth of insight for this life and our relationship with Him. This wouldn't be so that we could become puffed up and smarter than others. It would be so that we could have a greater level of relationship with Him. How many mental health problems would we avoid if only we had knowledge and insight to discern what was best before we made a decision?

This isn't to say that reading Scripture or knowing God are sure ways out of our depression and anxiety—that's not how it works. But we can learn and grow and improve the way we handle anxiety, and having a depth of knowledge of God and intimacy with Him helps immensely with that. This is the "top-down" approach that Paul emphasized in his prayer. Know God, and you will better know and understand yourself and the hardships and struggles and triggers you experience.

Top-down thinking is not just spiritual but also scientific. The middle part of our brain is where our emotions are formed. When things don't go our way, when there's a fork in the road, when we have to make a decision, we experience emotion. Sometimes we experience *a lot* of emotion—like when we're in the path of a bear. Other times we experience a *little* emotion, like when the bear is behind a fence at a zoo, but it's still glaring and growling at us. We react differently based on the situation. But when our emotions determine what we do next, that's bottom-up thinking.

Again, what we want is top-down thinking. The part of our brain related to intelligence and analysis is up top, near the front. This part is called the frontal cortex, and it's where we think and reason and determine, "What's the wise thing to do in this situation?" This is the part of the brain that should be in control. It's best when the reasoning part of the brain informs the emotional part of the brain so that our actions are intentional and controlled, and so that we can discern, process, and make logical choices, not overly emotional ones.

(As we wrote earlier, emotions, in themselves, are not "bad." They are God-given and important for our relationships and life. But when they dominate our choices and behavior, we can make unhelpful or harmful decisions and build patterns of anxiety.)

With top-down thinking, from a spiritual perspective, the goal is for every decision to be pure and blameless before Jesus, and the best way to do this is to act *in Him*. Our fruit of righteousness comes from only one place, one Person, and that's Jesus. Remember Hebrews 10:14: *"For by one sacrifice he has made* [not *will* make] *perfect forever those who are being made holy* [those who are being transformed into the image of Jesus]." The author of Hebrews goes on to talk about how this transformation doesn't come about by our acts of righteousness but by the fruit of righteousness developing in us. Hebrews 12:11 reminds us, *"No discipline seems pleasant at the time, but painful. Later on, however, it produces a harvest of righteousness and peace* ["*the peaceful fruit of righteousness*" ESV] *for those who have been trained by it."*

That's what all this knowledge and wisdom and discernment is for—to get us into that peaceful, non-anxiety-producing "*fruit of righteousness.*" It's to help our algorithm become reflexive. As our love for Jesus increases, we will know Him more, and knowing Jesus more will allow us to depend on Him to produce the fruit in us that glorifies Him.

As you pursue this transformative process, you'll find, in the beginning, that your steps will be very intentional. You'll have to think about almost every action, and you'll have to be mindful of using a top-down approach. But we promise you that as you learn more and more about Jesus—through reading His Word, memorizing Scripture, praying, being around other strong believers, reading helpful books, and listening to sermons—you'll begin to realize that those little steps you've been taking toward Him are more productive for developing that peaceful fruit of righteousness in your life than all of the steps that you used to take away from Him.

Yes, all those times when you did what you wanted—those times when you sought your own desires and opted for the thing that was an easy fix—do not compare to what you will experience when you commit to taking small, consistent steps toward Jesus. And, friend, it gets easier and easier. The first weeks and perhaps months will take a lot of intentionality on your part. They will require that you dig in and address some things that might be painful—maybe it's the way you spend your time or the way you engage with God. But each day spent pursuing this process will bring you closer to being reflexive in your walk with God, where abiding in Him comes as naturally as breathing. Before you know it, abiding in Christ will be your natural solution to handling stress, which will prevent it from causing you to become anxious.

When you have deeper insight into who God is and what His love is, then it changes the way you define and experience love. No human being loves perfectly, but, on top of that, as we discussed earlier in this book, our upbringing and life experiences alter the way we give and receive love.

Each of us has our own definition of love. Those of us who grew up under performance-based rules tend to bring that mindset into our relationship with God. We think that we need to earn God's love, but, even more than that, we often present God as performance-based to others, too. We judge or evaluate non-Christians based on their actions, on what they do or don't do. You don't see Jesus doing this anywhere in Scripture—He was always most concerned with people's hearts, not their actions—but we do this to each other. We size one another up based on our performance, and we make judgments.

Jesus was never condemning to those who came to Him earnestly. All He did was show love to people. When we adopt a similar mindset—that love is in abundance, and it is for everyone regardless of their performance—that's when we will realize that we don't have to fix anyone. We don't have to police anyone. We don't have to convince anyone to believe or think a certain way. We just have to love. And that is the kind of insight we receive from top-down praying.

In the next chapter, we will continue to look at relationship lessons from the book of Philippians. We'll further see how they can enhance our spiritual and emotional health, and enable us to better put the algorithm into practice as we address our anxiety, stress, and fear.

WELLNESS EXERCISE: GENOGRAM AND SPIRITUAL TIMELINE

There is a tool that we use a lot in therapy called a genogram. It's a type of family tree, but it allows you to be very detailed in the way that you portray family relationships and generational patterns, which can help you to understand how your family history has affected the way you think and react. You can go to a website such as genopro.com/genogram/ and learn how to create your own genogram. I (James) highly encourage you to do so. Here are some exercises to assist you in this process.

Think through your family heritage. (If you are someone who has a history of abuse, this family tree exercise might be very difficult for you, so let us be clear: you don't have to participate. You can move to the next exercise if your past is too troubling for you to think about right now. This other exercise is to think through your spiritual timeline, which we describe three paragraphs down.)

Who were the people around you while you were growing up, and what were they like? What were their struggles? How did those struggles impact you? How did these family members and others influence you and treat you? The goal in this exercise is not to blame or accuse but to gain new insights that will inform how you approach life and relationships. For example, if you grew up with an angry father, then, as an adult, you might be triggered by angry people. Knowing how your feelings are connected to the past is very helpful for realizing that, in your reactions to people and events, you're not silly or even "crazy," as some people might say.

Triggers are real, and they happen for real reasons. They're built into us biologically and psychologically, and they are very attached to that fight-or-flight system we've talked about. At their basic level, triggers are there to try to help us stay safe and protect ourselves. But when it comes to emotional triggers, as we get older, and especially as we develop in spiritual maturity, Jesus wants to come in and help heal our emotions. It's not that triggers are necessarily bad or wrong, but there is a better way. Real freedom can be found through Christ. This is why it's important to invite Jesus into your family history—your family baggage, if you will.

Next, think through your spiritual timeline. Remember that, in the Old Testament, God would intervene in the lives of the Israelites, and when He moved in a mighty way, they would build altars or monuments to remember what He did. (See, for example, Genesis 35:1–7; Joshua 4:1–9.) Every time they saw a certain monument, they would remember a specific act of God that had saved them from something horrible and insurmountable from a human perspective.

When you look back on your life so far, what were some big moments when God showed up? Identify those times and find a way to mark them with an "altar" or "monument" to keep them present in your thoughts. Each of us can hopefully identify certain instances when God intervened in some way, and it can be encouraging and helpful to remember those times. Take some time to think about and write down what comes to mind. How might these memories influence your algorithm focal points?

17

BUILDING STRONG RELATIONSHIPS, PART 2

Lessons 4–7 from Paul's letter to the church in Philippi help us to build stronger relationships with God and other people and to enter into the peace God desires for us.

RELATIONSHIP LESSONS FROM PHILIPPIANS

Lesson 4: Know That God Is in Control

And because of my chains, most of the brothers and sisters have become confident in the Lord and dare all the more to proclaim the gospel without fear. (Philippians 1:14)

Fear and anxiety trick us into thinking that life should be a certain way, and any path other than the path that brings us the most comfort is a path to be fearful and anxious about. Paul shows us a different way.

Most people would agree that Paul's being in prison was not an ideal situation. Some would also argue that it was unfair. Here was

Paul, doing the Lord's work, and what did he have to show for it? He was imprisoned.

But Paul and the Philippians didn't see it that way. No, Paul didn't like being in prison, but what he could not deny was how God had used Paul's chains to turn people's hearts toward Him! This is why perspective matters. Paul and the church at Philippi turned a very scary, potentially anxiety-producing situation into one that God could use for His glory. They took the stress that Paul's chains certainly created and surrendered it to the Lord. They took something horrible and, instead of worrying and fretting and becoming fearful or depressed over it, gave it to God—and God showed up.

We see another example of this perspective in the book of Acts. The disciples were beaten and pushed down, but they came away from that experience praising God all the more, thankful that they were worthy of such hardship in the name of Christ! (See Acts 5:17–41.) This incredible mindset was present throughout the early church. They saw the blessings that came from chains. They saw how stress could improve their spiritual growth. And people came to know Christ because of it. The disciples' stress caused them to move closer to God, not away from Him.

This is an important dynamic, because we tend to think, "If only I can get this obstacle out of my path, *then* I'll be able to fully give everything to God," or "If only I can overcome these chains, *then* I can be at my best for Jesus!" But, many times, it's the chains and the obstacles that push us closer to God—putting us in a position where we can rest in Him in the midst of our difficulties.

In His teachings, Jesus flipped everything on its head. In His Sermon on the Mount in Matthew 5, He taught concepts that don't come naturally to us—concepts such as these:

+ Finding joy in suffering (see verses 11–12)
+ Turning the other cheek (see verses 38–39)
+ Giving someone more than what they want to take from you (see verse 40)

- Walking two miles for someone instead of one (also called "going the extra mile") (see verse 41)
- Loving your enemy (see verses 43–44)

These are difficult responses to master, and they require help from the Holy Spirit. So, how do we get started on the right path? What does it look like to take that first intentional step to living a sacrificial life that acknowledges God is in control?

For each of these teachings (and for many more), the best thing—once again—is to take two steps back:

When something happens in life that is unpleasant, before you react, take two steps back.

When someone wrongs you, when someone takes from you, when people ask for a favor that feels overwhelming, when life is unfair, don't react—take two steps back.

Pausing and stepping away from the moment will allow you to engage the algorithm, abide in the presence of God, and pursue top-down thinking. It will allow you to go from asking, "How do I fix this?" or "How do I win in this situation?" to asking, "How can God be glorified in this circumstance?" and "What would be the loving thing in this situation?

I (Ronnie) remember a time when my daughter Emily was in the sixth grade, starting into those wonderful teenage years. Emily walked through the dining room, where I was seated at one end of the table, farthest from the doorway, and my wife, Anne, Emily's mother, was at the other end. Now, Emily was a very compliant child. She never complained, and she was always eager to help. But, this time, as Emily was passing through the room, and Anne said something to her, I saw Emily's eye roll from across the room! She sarcastically said, "Whatever" and continued on her way upstairs, even slamming the bedroom door behind her.

Anne was furious. I thought she was going to climb across the table! "Are you going to let her get away with that?" she said to me. So, I pumped the brakes and took two steps back.

We had always prayed that our children would love God and that they would have God's heart—that God would act in them and help them to increase in wisdom and stature and in favor with God and man. (See Luke 2:52.) "Let's give God a chance," I said.

So Anne and I held hands and prayed. Five minutes later, Emily came back downstairs and apologized.

If we had run up there and punished her, we might have "fixed it," but we would have missed out on allowing God to do a work in Emily's heart. When we let God do His thing, wonderful results can happen. Not only that, but we will also have less anxiety in our lives and relationships because we will have relinquished this pressure we have to fix things.

You can try your best to change somebody's attitude, but it's not going to work. Only God can do that through the person of His Spirit and the power of His Word. (See Hebrews 4:12.)

Lesson 5: Live with Right Priorities

But what does it matter? The important thing is that in every way, whether from false motives or true, Christ is preached. And because of this I rejoice. Yes, and I will continue to rejoice, for I know that through your prayers and God's provision of the Spirit of Jesus Christ what has happened to me will turn out for my deliverance. (Philippians 1:18–19)

When you signed on as a Christian, you stepped into the kingdom of God. You left your own kingdom behind to enter into what God is building and the work He is doing. But it's still so easy to seek our own kingdoms, isn't it?

God wants us to live a great life, a blessed life. He just wants to make sure we have our priorities right and understand that His kingdom comes first. You see, when we put God's kingdom first, then James's kingdom and Ronnie's kingdom and your kingdom will automatically be taken care of! It's when we get things upside down, when we put our kingdoms first, that our anxiety and depression often go through the roof, threatening our peace and our effectiveness in life. We need to have the right priorities.

Relinquishing control to God is not going to be easy. You will experience internal friction. But that feeling of friction, that feeling of resistance, happens because the "what-ifs" are going off in your brain. Few statements are more anxiety-producing than those that begin with "What if...?": "What if it doesn't work out?" "What if I don't like what God does?" "What if I lose something important to me?" "What if this affects my life in a bad way?" "What if this is painful?" "What if...?"

We worry about what-ifs, but God is the I Am.

I (Ronnie) remember when a friend called saying that he had needed my prayers the day before. "Okay, I'll pray for you now," I said. He shrugged it off because the thing he needed prayer for had come and gone. I insisted, "I'll pray for you today, and God will hear it yesterday. He is the great I Am. He's not limited by time or space."

We get so caught up in the tomorrows, but when we stay focused on what *might* happen, we take control back from God. He is here—now—with you, and He wants you fully present with Him. Again, you may feel resistant when you start these intentional steps, but that is because you're human. The more you practice them, the more you'll find that you can trust God with tomorrow.

In Philippians 1:20, Paul writes, *"I eagerly expect and hope that I will in no way be ashamed, but will have sufficient courage so that now as always Christ will be exalted in my body, whether by life or by death."* Paul's use of the word *"eagerly"* shows that he had an eternal perspective—he had a passion for what God would do. This is where we tend to get hung up. We aren't passionate about God's perspective. He sees and knows and understands so much more than we do, yet we think that our way is better! When we can adopt a passion for God's perspective, it becomes much easier to give Him control.

Lesson 6: Put Others First

I will continue with all of you for your progress and joy in the faith. (Philippians 1:25)

Who we are is connected to who we live and work with. The progress and success we experience personally will directly impact the progress and success we experience as a family, church, team, and so forth. This is why it's not just about you and your success or me and my success. It's about how our combined growth and change and breakthrough will help others.

If you've ever been on a team with a really great player, then you already understand this concept. There's a sense that even if you don't perform at your best, the team still has a chance because there's a star player who will carry everyone to victory.

In our spiritual lives, the star player is the Holy Spirit. He makes us better. As you fight your anxiety, you're not just doing it for yourself. You're doing it for your family, your kids, and your community, and you can ask the Holy Spirit to encourage and guide you. Keeping the bigger picture in mind can be motivating as you do the hard, intentional steps of working through the algorithm and learning to abide in Christ.

Lesson 7: Behavior Is an Important Indicator

Whatever happens, conduct yourself in a manner worthy of the gospel of Christ. (Philippians 1:27)

We have talked about developing our spiritual fruit. Another word we might use for *fruit* is *behavior*. Way back when I (Ronnie) was in elementary school, students received a "conduct grade." My mom was always quick to look at my conduct grade because it represented what others thought of our family. My conduct in school reflected who we were at home.

Our actions and behavior—the way we live life, how we handle struggles, how we treat others, and how we respond to the good and the bad that happens to us—are what the world sees. Our behavior is a good indication of the quality of our fruit and what's going on in our lives, and it's also a representation of our spiritual family.

My (Ronnie's) dear friend Johnny grew up in a different environment than I did, and the language he used was not always edifying. He cussed a lot and used some pretty crass sayings. One day, he expressed to me that he had become convicted about this but didn't know how to stop. So, we prayed, and I gave him some Scriptures to keep in his pocket. I told him that, when he got ready to say something he shouldn't, he should grab hold of his leg near his pocket. I wanted him to feel that paper there, where Scripture was speaking truth into his life.

So, he did it. He'd get talking and then grab his leg when he felt he needed some extra help. It got to the point where people were laughing about it! But his cussing stopped.

Johnny has had to overcome many such behaviors over the years as he is molded in the way of Christ, and he is the first to tell you that it is not his own might or willpower that has allowed him to change his behavior and his life. It's only Jesus. Only Jesus can do the work. And as love, joy, peace, patience, kindness, goodness, faithfulness, gentleness, and self-control come forth from you, too, the world will take notice because of how different you will be.

HELP, IT'S NOT WORKING!

We can implement these truths and exercise our faith and take intentional steps in our communities and relationships, but what happens when we feel that our efforts are far outpacing the results that we see? This is when, again, it's important to take a few steps back.

Most of us approach life thinking that our results should be on par with the amount of effort that we put in. So if we put in 50 percent effort, we should see an improvement by 50 percent.

But this isn't how life works.

When we first begin putting in effort, we usually don't see much of a result, if any. In fact, things might actually become worse—or seem worse—for a time. But as our efforts continue and build as time passes, then we suddenly see the results boost, seemingly out of nowhere! The important thing is to stick with it and not let yourself fall victim to the "I quit" zone.

A great example of this "effort versus results curve,"[32] is when someone actively tries to lose weight. Many people can lose five pounds relatively easily. Unfortunately, though, when most people lose five pounds, they end up gaining ten pounds back. This causes their results to drop far below their expectations, and that's when many people give up or decide that a particular diet or lifestyle isn't helpful for them. But when people persist, when they hang on even if the results aren't favorable, the outcomes may eventually outperform their expectations.

Let us say again that there is nothing easy about being conformed to the image of Jesus. There's nothing easy about taking intentional steps to combat anxiety and fear. There's nothing easy about turning your life on its head and saying, "I'm doing things differently from now on." But there also isn't any shame in the process. Remember, when a child falls down while learning to walk, there's no shame in that. And God is right there with you, cheering you on, as your small steps turn into great steps.

As you go through this process, you'll still feel anxious. You may have doubt. You might not feel as though you can give it all over to God quite yet, and you might have major unease when it comes to fully entering into Christian community the way God intended. But keep taking those steps toward Him and others. To change your life and outlook, you need the help of a supportive church community. You cannot do it alone, but in order to do it effectively, you must communicate well, and that's what we'll cover in the next chapter.

---

32. Seth Godin, *The Dip* (New York: Penguin Random House, 2007); Seth Godin, Seth's Blog, https://seths.blog/2007/05/images_from_the/; Navin Kabra, "Understanding the Dip," FutureIQ, https://futureiq.substack.com/p/understanding-the-dip.

WELLNESS EXERCISE: MAKE GRATITUDE YOUR ATTITUDE!

A number of research studies have shown that practicing gratitude is very helpful in several ways.[33] Various passages in the Bible affirm the blessings of being grateful and thankful. (See, for example, Philippians 4:6–7; Colossians 2:6–7; 3:14–16.) Focusing on what you have to be thankful for can help you emotionally, it can help you to build stronger relationships, and it can help you see the silver lining that God is with you, no matter what you might be going through, and He is sovereign in your life.

For example, if there is someone in your life who represents an "enemy," someone who is very bothersome, what if you wrote down a few reasons why you could be grateful that God has placed them in your life? My (James's) grandfather used to say that God puts some people in your life for no other reason than to build your character.

---

33. Geyze Diniz et al., "The Effects of Gratitude Interventions: A Systematic Review and Meta-Analysis," Einstein journal (São Paulo) 2023;21:eRW0371, https://journal.einstein.br/article/the-effects-of-gratitude-interventions-a-systematic-review-and-meta-analysis/.

So, you might say that so-and-so is in your life to help you be more patient, kind, or humble. This is something to be thankful for.

Keeping a gratitude journal, a notebook where you write down a few things each day you can be thankful for, is another great practice. If you find yourself anxious or stressed throughout the day, it is much easier to intentionally remember what you are grateful for if you began your morning by writing down a few of those things. Make sure you regularly pray and thank God for His goodness in your life and for giving you the things you are grateful for.

Another gratitude practice is to write a letter to someone who has blessed you. Perhaps you had a recent conversation with them that left you feeling encouraged. Maybe you want to thank a godly grade-school teacher whose impact has stuck with you. Maybe you want to encourage your parent by expressing how much you appreciate their influence in your life and the sacrifices they have made for you over the years. Write a letter once a month or so to someone who is special to you, someone for whom you are grateful. This will no doubt be very encouraging for them to receive, but it will also help you to remember how God has put these people in your life and how their presence has blessed and benefitted you.

You may also need to write a letter of forgiveness to someone as a means of helping you to heal emotionally and/or as a potential step in healing a relationship. Forgiving others can be very difficult. As Christians, we are not to keep a tally of those who have wronged us and how they hurt us. (See, for example, Matthew 18:21–22; 1 Corinthians 13:4–5.) Jesus demonstrated this better than anyone because He was always quick to forgive others. The truth is that forgiveness is just as much, if not more, for the person forgiving as it is for the person being forgiven. There is a freedom awaiting those who forgive others. Here is how forgiving others can lead you into gratitude: As Christians, we experienced the ultimate forgiveness when we chose to become followers of Jesus. Jesus took our place and received our penalty on the cross. Forgiving others reminds us of what Jesus did for us, which is something that we should be tremendously grateful for.

18

REDUCING ANXIETY THROUGH EFFECTIVE COMMUNICATION

At the end of Philippians 3, Paul talked about how we are citizens of heaven, not of earth, and so we won't always fit in here. We're almost like ambassadors—inviting people to learn more about the kingdom of God.

It's from this perspective that Paul wrote about loving and longing for his dear friends in Philippi. This relationship between Paul and the Philippians wasn't the casual friendship that we see in many churches today. It was significant to Paul because he wasn't doing very well. He was in prison, and he didn't know if he would be released or if he would die there.

For Paul to write about loving and longing for these people, the Philippians must have provided him with an emotional support system that helped to sustain him in his suffering. We know that it was the Philippians who sent Epaphroditus to Paul in order to help meet Paul's needs. That particular strategy hadn't worked out the way everyone had hoped due to Epaphroditus's illness, and Paul ended up sending him back. However, from this example, we can see how invested the Philippian church was in Paul's emotional, mental, and physical well-being, despite the distance between them.

The relationships that impact us can be from either our past or our present, and from within our home or church or from thousands of miles away. God works through relationships in such a powerful way that even the memory of a prior strong relationship can be enough to support and encourage us. (You might have used memories of past relationships when building your algorithm!) But for a relationship to be established and flourish in the way God intended, there needs to be good communication between the parties.

COMMUNICATION BASICS

It's a bit mind-blowing that children can move through the process of obtaining a full education, from kindergarten through high school, without having to take a single interpersonal relations class. They might be taught how to give speeches or how to make a presentation at a meeting, but they aren't often taught simple relational communication.

Communication is the bedrock of any relationship—and our anxiety, our stress, and our fears all affect the way we communicate. But by knowing and practicing the principles of good communication, you can become more effective and lower your anxiety when it comes to interacting with others. You can also develop deep, meaningful relationships that bring you joy—the kind of relationships that Paul experienced and relied on in his darkest times. Just think about what it would mean for you to have people you could go to—people who would love you and speak truth into your life—when your anxious thoughts have gotten out of hand, and you're in a spiral. There are many good resources available on developing good communication skills, from podcasts to articles to books.[34]

---

34. See, for example, John C. Maxwell, *Everyone Communicates, Few Connect: What the Most Effective People Do Differently* (Nashville, TN: Thomas Nelson, 2010).

Know Your Communication Strengths and Weaknesses

It all starts by knowing what kind of a communicator you are. One way to go about this is to check with people you know and trust. Ask them if they think you're good at communication or if you need to grow in this area. Ask where your shortcomings are, what they've noticed that you could improve upon, and so on. Getting these insights into how others perceive your communication style might be hard to hear, but it is so helpful for taking steps toward change. A word of warning: if you want an honest answer, you cannot become defensive and cut the other person off by trying to explain away your poor communication habits. This is why you should be sure to ask someone you trust who is not going to be overly critical and whose insights you are more willing to receive.

Become an Active Listener

But great communication doesn't just involve the words you use and how you use them. It also requires great listening.

Most of us think we know how to listen, but, more often than not, when someone makes a statement, we're immediately thinking about our response to it—not about what the person has said. And when we *do* focus on what the other person is saying, we tend to jump in and interrupt. We want to respond quickly, *but that isn't listening*.

A bedrock of communication is what's called "active listening." We tend to think of listening as something passive, but active listening requires a lot of intentionality. Often, it necessitates putting your phone away and limiting distractions. It requires using eye contact and nonverbal cues, such as head nods, that indicate you are paying attention and invested in what the other person is saying.

To listen well, you have to be motivated. You must be devoted to the listening process for the sake of the other person. When you engage in active listening with someone, you will find that it will change the way that person responds to you, because it will show that you value them. It will tell them that they are important to you, and when someone feels important within a relationship, they are much more likely to put in the hard work to make the relationship thrive. This concept is especially essential for parents of teenagers to understand.

Once you've fully listened to someone and given them the time and space to share what's on their heart, then you can practice what is called "reflection." This is when you reflect back to the person what you have heard them say. Reflection is a common approach with therapists. I (James) will listen to someone share what's going on in their life, and then, when they are finished, I will reiterate what I heard them express, but I attach a feeling to it. So, for example, if they share with me a situation in which a friend hasn't gotten back to them regarding an important matter, I might reflect with, "So, what I'm hearing you say is that you're confused about why your friend has been so distant." By attaching a feeling (in this example, the feeling of confusion) to the situation, I'm helping both them and me to better understand what they want and what they are hoping for in the situation.

A more basic version of reflection can be used in relationships that are very strained. I've worked with family members who were having trouble getting along with one another, and their assignment was simply to state to one another what they are feeling and why. They might say something like, "I feel unloved because you never spend time with me," or "I feel frustrated that you are on your phone so much." The person receiving that statement must repeat it back to them: "I hear you say that you feel unloved because I don't spend time with you," or "I hear you say that you are frustrated because of how much time I spend on my phone." It's the most foundational way to get opposing people to communicate. As this process is repeated, with one person making a statement, and their family member responding reflectively, true communication can occur, because it eliminates accusations or statements that begin with, "Well, you...." It can completely shift the way in which the two people communicate, helping them to move on from arguing with one another because their focus is now on repairing the relationship.

A similar method works for people who are dealing with anxiety, especially social anxiety. By having a template to follow, they can communicate what they are feeling and why. In therapy, we might help them develop a script they can memorize for starting a conversation or for everyday back-and-forth exchanges with their acquaintances. For example, I (James) may ask them to memorize the following sequence of questions and statements: "How are you today?" "Did you do anything fun last weekend?" "What are you working on at your job?" "I'm glad I ran into you. I need to get to my next appointment, but it was great to see you. Hope to talk with you again soon." You may have noticed that each of these remarks can be stated regardless of how the other person responds. We also usually plan for contingencies, such as if the person responds by asking if *they* did anything fun over the weekend. I always remind my clients that no one knows more about their life than they do. So, they can simply say that they did not do anything noteworthy over the weekend or describe the fun thing they did, and then return to the script.

In therapy, much of what we do is simply listen closely and help people understand how they truly feel. When we do that well, our hope is that they will leave feeling heard and having a better understanding of their emotions and a clearer understanding of why they feel the way they do. When this happens, the person is usually able to think of solutions for their problems. This result is striking when you think about it! Most people don't need advice or solutions. Most people need to be heard, and then they can take what they learn through being heard and having someone respond to them reflectively, and they can implement change on their own.

Ask Clarifying Questions

Third, great listeners ask clarifying questions. When we're listening, and something doesn't add up or doesn't make sense, it's important to ask questions that draw out the information we need to fully understand the situation. For example, if a friend is telling you about how stressful his job is and all of the deadlines that he is under, it would be easy to assume that his main problem is the job itself. But by asking clarifying questions, you might discover that the *real* issue is with his boss and how the boss manages workflow. Clarifying questions allow you to truly understand a situation so that you can fully engage in conversation about it.

Helping someone feel heard in this way is more powerful than you can imagine. Jesus's interactions with struggling people always seemed to help them feel understood and valued. Think about His interactions with the woman at the well (see John 4:4–30), the adulterous woman (see John 8:1–11), Zacchaeus the tax collector (see Luke 19:1–10), and the woman with the issue of blood (see, for example, Mark 5:25–34). Helping someone feel heard and accepted despite how others may see them or what they may have done is something Jesus wants all of us to model, just as He did for us.

Slow Down to Be Present with People

All of the previous communication basics we've discussed are good and important, but communication can still break down if we don't take the time to *be present with people*. Dallas Willard, who was a philosopher, professor, and all-around amazing theologian, once responded to someone who asked him how to live a balanced and effective life by saying that he needed to "ruthlessly eliminate hurry" from his life.[35]

Take a minute to let that idea soak in.

"Busy" is a state of the body, but "hurry" is a state of the mind. When we eliminate the mental pressure of hurry, we can be physically busy but mentally at peace. We can have a full schedule but not be frazzled and stressed out.

---

35. John Mark Comer, *The Ruthless Elimination of Hurry* (Colorado Springs, CO: Waterbrook, 2019), 18–19.

When we're busy, we make time for what's important. We prioritize our time. But when we're in a hurry, we don't seem to have any time for anyone or anything. See the difference?

We live in a society that prizes accomplishment and efficiency. While there is nothing inherently wrong with these outcomes, it goes against the grain for us humans to prioritize being productive with our time but leave the results up to God.

Some years ago, I (Ronnie) was always notoriously late. By the time I met with my last patient of the day, it was well past that patient's appointment time. I just could not keep things on schedule, and, as a result, I'd be rushing across town after work and blowing into the church parking lot thirty or forty minutes after a meeting that I was scheduled to be a part of had started.

One of those times, I was rushing up the stairs to get to the meeting room, taking the steps two at a time, when I tripped and fell back to the landing. In that moment, I had this thought of Jesus running up the stairs of the temple two at a time, His robe flapping behind him.

And suddenly I felt convicted.

I don't think Jesus ever took steps two at a time, because Jesus was never in a hurry. Despite His being in high demand, and His to-do list being one of the most important in the history of the world, Jesus paced Himself. He didn't have to hurry because His mind was at peace, and He understood His priorities through His relationship with the Father.

Develop Empathy for Others

Therefore, my brothers and sisters, you whom I love and long for, my joy and crown, stand firm in the Lord in this way, dear friends! (Philippians 4:1)

When James was younger, he loved to drive off-road trucks. He'd take them through the mud and the countryside and really put them to the test. I (Ronnie) thought it would be good for us to fix up an old truck that he could take out and do whatever he wanted with. He could off-road it as much as he liked, and it wouldn't matter because it would be his. So, I asked a bunch of my friends for leads on used trucks, and I ended up finding an old Bronco a few hours north of our hometown. The only problem with the Bronco was that it didn't run!

One of our family friends hauled the truck down closer to where we lived so we could work on it with a gifted mechanic in south Mississippi. Every weekend, James and I would drive about sixty miles to work on it with the mechanic. We'd sleep in the back of our Chevy Suburban, and then we'd drive home on Saturday evening to be ready for church the next day. I had big expectations for this time with my son. I thought for sure we'd be able to bond and grow closer, but, as the weeks went by, it was clear that the opposite was happening. Our relationship was getting worse.

I went straight to God. "What is going on, Lord?" I asked. Almost immediately, I felt God say, "You talk too much, Ronnie."

And He was right. I would spend all of the two hours in the car, there and back, talking. I would fill every quiet moment with more and more words, and the Spirit convicted me that it was time for me to be quiet and listen.

On our next trip, I just sat there. The silence was killing me, but I waited and prayed. We didn't talk the whole way there or for most of the ride back. Then, about five miles from home, James asked, "Dad, can I ask you something?"

I almost drove us off the road, I was so excited!

He asked me about something that was going on at school, but instead of giving advice, I asked him what he thought he should do about it. He explained his thoughts, and all I did was reassure him that he was on the right track, that he was seeing the situation clearly.

Later, he told his mom that it was the best trip we had ever had.

I needed to shut my mouth and see things from James's perspective for the sake of our relationship. That is what it means to have empathy, and it is key to having a solid relationship.

Some people are not going to talk if you don't give them the space to do so. My (James's) personality is that of a peacemaker, and I'm pretty quiet in a group. My dad is more of a take-charge, leader type. If he fills the space with words and conversation, then I don't usually feel much of a need to speak up.

Exercising empathy means putting yourself in someone else's shoes. You try to understand what they're thinking and feeling, what life must be like for them. Empathy is like sympathy but with compassion and relatability. Empathy is when you understand why a person feels the way they feel, and it moves you.

Empathy requires self-awareness. The more you understand your own feelings and what causes them, the better you will be able to listen to and empathize with others.

Our experiences create a lens through which we see ourselves, others, and the world. We interpret everything through this lens, but the tricky part is that no two people's lenses are the same. We each have a unique way of seeing the world and our interactions within it. But despite seeing life differently, we each also have access to the same emotions.

When we have empathy in our relationships, we are able to understand the feelings of others so that we can enter into whatever it is they're going through. We can sit with someone in their frustration or pain or hopelessness and think of times when we were frustrated or pained or hopeless. Again, the circumstances might have been very different, but the emotions are similar.

When a woman comes in for grief counseling because she has suffered a miscarriage, it would be easy for me (James) to say, "I can't relate to that. I'm a man, so my life experience is very different." But while I can't relate to that specific experience, I *can* relate to strong feelings of grief and loss. I can relate to the guilt that she may be putting on herself, thinking that she has done something wrong.

Empathy therefore allows us to use emotion to connect with others and share in their pain and struggle, even though their life experiences may be very different from our own. Where we tend to get it wrong is when we make it all about us.

A friend might express their anguish over the fact that they have just lost their job, and, as good empathizers, our minds may jump to when we worked for an untrustworthy company or when we were laid off during the COVID-19 pandemic. Instead of channeling that memory to allow us to access those emotions and feelings, we are tempted to start talking about our own experiences. Before we know it, we've taken over the conversation, giving details about our own job issues and past job stresses.

While it was supposed to be about the other person, we made it about us. When this happens, we take something from the person who tried to share with us. You've likely had this happen to you. It is not only frustrating, but it also causes you to feel dismissed rather than valued.

A much better way to use our experiences in empathy is not to first share our own stories but rather draw on our experiences to say things like, "Wow, that must have made you feel unappreciated," or "Has going through that experience caused you to wonder about the value you bring to your work?"

As the conversation goes on, you can reveal that you have been in a similar position, but empathy is about keeping the spotlight on the person who is hurting, the person who is dealing with a lot at that moment.

Recognize the Spiritual Opposition

I plead with Euodia and I plead with Syntyche to be of the same mind in the Lord. (Philippians 4:2)

Despite Paul's incredible relationship with the church at Philippi, the believers in that church didn't always get along, as we see from this verse. What's even more surprising is that these women who were causing a stir weren't casual church members. They were prominent members who had walked with Paul and worked with him. (See verse 3.)

There will be times of struggle in all relationships. Relationships are hard, but it seems that family and church relationships are the hardest. This is because they mean the most to us.

Jesus's prayer in John 17 was for unity in the church. He saw the disunity among His followers, He saw the infighting and issues, and He laid the groundwork for a better way. Jesus preached about the importance of love above all else, telling us, *"As I have loved you, so you must love one another"* (John 13:34).

It is this love that Satan is determined to mess up.

When we're in conflict with someone, it's easy to think of them as the enemy. It's easy to feel that if *that* person could just change or leave, everything would get better. But when we feel this way, we're missing the big picture. The person might be causing mischief and trouble, but, ultimately, they are not the enemy, and they are not the one whom we need to fight. It is Satan and his forces that we are up against. (See Ephesians 6:12.) When we understand this and begin to put the blame on Satan, where it belongs, we might find our hearts soften toward the people with whom we were so frustrated before.

We must realize that Satan seeks to cause problems within relationships. We think that our anxiety is caused by traffic jams, pressure on our jobs, daily stress, or our hurried schedules, but it may be that we are experiencing anxiety because the enemy is wreaking havoc in our relationships.

Paul saw that the Philippian church was being threatened by the relationship problems between Euodia and Syntyche. He knew that this conflict could cause a lot of damage to the work being done there. His challenge to these women was to get in line, to set their minds on what was important. He knew that if they both focused on things above instead of the relational issues between them, their relationship would improve.

To have the mind of Christ, we must "empty ourselves," like Jesus did. He emptied Himself of His heavenly position and became a servant. He left His glory behind and came to earth to show us God's love. When we focus on the solution, not the problem, we redirect our minds to pursue the things that we really want rather than the things that we don't want or the things that are causing us struggle. Jesus kept His mind on things above, not letting the squabbles between His disciples get Him down (think about that!). Paul asked these women to do the same. He was asking them to set their disagreements aside and focus on their common goal of growing the church and spreading the gospel.

Think about the people whom you struggle with, the people whom you believe cause you anxiety. Is the message in this chapter one you need to receive? What freedom might you experience by realizing that your anxiety and problems are not caused by flesh and blood but by the spiritual darkness we can't see? And how might this change your algorithm and the way you focus on what is true, noble, right, pure, lovely, admirable, excellent, and praiseworthy?

THE WAY GOD INTENDED

People in healthy relationships communicate their feelings and needs. As much as possible, they address issues quickly and effectively. When they can't do that, they set aside their differences and focus on the common goal. People in healthy relationships make time for one another. Listening is key, and love is the goal. Those who are in healthy relationships also "see" one another—they see when someone is hurting or struggling or in need of a listening ear. Healthy relationships prioritize people over hurry, and they practice empathy.

As we expressed earlier, having healthy relationships is crucial to working through our fear and anxiety, because these relationships help to remind us that we aren't alone. There is wisdom in having a multitude of counselors (see Proverbs 11:14; 15:22), and this is true not only when it comes to big life decisions but also to mental struggles that are getting the best of us. And healthy relationships help us to remember that people are not our enemies. Satan is, and when relationships get tough, he is the one at which to point our finger.

At the beginning of part 3 of this book, we said that it might seem odd talking about relationships in a book about anxiety. Hopefully, you can now see that nothing could be less strange. Scientific studies have overwhelmingly shown that relationships are critical to our wellness. Dr. Robert Waldinger, the current director of a long-running Harvard study, stated, "The people who were the most satisfied in their relationships at age 50 were the healthiest at age 80."[36]

It really is amazing that science is confirming what the Bible has said for two thousand years. Being in relationship with other people is important. Relationships are part of God's plan for our wholeness and happiness. We must learn how to communicate and be in relationship with people if we're going to tackle our anxiety and fully experience the presence of God.

Healthy relationships go hand in hand with living a Christlike life—but what does such a life mean in practical terms? What does it look like as our anxiety lessens and we're able to operate from a place of abiding in Christ? We'll cover this in the next chapter as we move to part 4, "The Algorithm and Our Wellness."

---

36. Robert Waldinger, quoted in Liz Mineo, "Good Genes Are Nice, but Joy Is Better," *The Harvard Gazette*, April 11, 2017, https://news.harvard.edu/gazette/story/2017/04/over-nearly-80-years-harvard-study-has-been-showing-how-to-live-a-healthy-and-happy-life/.

WELLNESS EXERCISE: GOOD COMMUNICATION TECHNIQUES

Moving toward wellness means that we are always working to be better communicators. Take time to do some online research and become more familiar with healthy communication techniques, such as active listening, reflective statements, and conflict resolution.

Many of us tend to avoid conflict. The truth is that conflict is really an opportunity for intimacy and connection. Think about that last sentence. What if your usual experience of conflict was that you ran toward it when it occurred, rather than away from it, because it had the potential for you to feel a deeper sense of connection with others? Jesus spoke tough truths to people, but when He did, those who were open to receiving and who recognized His love and goodwill toward them felt seen rather than judged. If you approach conflict with the tools we discussed in chapter 18, you will be amazed at how well conflict can lead to your feeling connected and encouraged.

As previously suggested, ask someone you trust if you are a good communicator and a good listener. Write down their feedback, then ask someone else whom you trust. After asking a few people, really study what they had to say about you. Many of us are too insecure to do this. Don't be. None of us is born with good communication skills. And, remember, it is not as though most of us have had a class on how to be a good communicator. You don't have to feel ashamed or guilty if your friends offer pointed feedback on areas where you may need improvement.

Some practical questions you might ask are:

- Do you feel like I am a good listener?
- Do I have a tendency to make the conversation about me and what I am dealing with?
- When you share things with me, do you feel like I truly understand what you are telling me?
- Do I talk too much, without allowing you time to express your own thoughts and feelings?
- Am I someone you trust not to share things you have told me in confidence?
- Do I have any annoying habits that make it difficult to talk with me or to get along with me?
- When we talk, do I only try to "fix" your problems, or do you feel like I try to understand and encourage you?
- Are there people you would rather share your struggles with? (They do not need to be named.) If so, what makes them more approachable than I am?

Again, make sure that you are prepared to simply listen to the person's feedback. Make sure to take notes and compare what others say about you. The goal here is to have a growth mindset and not a fixed mindset. Thank the person for being vulnerable and sharing openly with you. Then, practice the areas that you see highlighted in your notes. Really work on getting better at communication. So many aspects of our insecurities and anxieties can be addressed by our becoming more comfortable with others.

Part Four:

THE ALGORITHM
AND LONG-TERM WELLNESS

19

A LIFE OF WELLNESS

The book of Philippians discusses several different pathways that lead to long-term wellness. The first is found in Philippians 4:9, where Paul says that we are to put into practice what we are learning. This is where we daily implement new rhythms and turn old patterns of worry and stress into new patterns of peace and joy.

But what happens when a crisis hits, and you're thrown completely off guard? Unanticipated emergency situations require a specific approach, and we call this path an "intervention." An intervention may also be needed at certain times in order to break a long-standing cycle of anxiety or fear.

A life of wellness balances both steady growth and intervention: we continue to pursue our daily wellness practices, but we also learn how to intervene when things get hard. Let's review the importance of building daily practices and strong relationships before we dive into what to do when intervention is needed.

FOUNDATIONS FOR DAILY PRACTICE

Daily practice is all about developing your relationship with God through Jesus, and your relationships with others. Philippians 2:1

reads, "*Therefore if you have any encouragement from being united with Christ, if any comfort from his love, if any common sharing in the Spirit, if any tenderness and compassion....*" We are to work on our relationship with Jesus, building it up; and, through it, His Spirit will flow out from us to others. This communal benefit will bring encouragement, comfort, love, tenderness, and compassion, impacting every person around us.

As we've mentioned, this doesn't happen unless we are abiding in Christ. People often ask, "How can I know if I'm fully loving God? How do I know I'm giving Him everything? How do I know I'm abiding in Christ and resting in His Spirit?"

So much of how we love God is tied to how we love the people around us. Again, when God is flowing through us, and we are extending compassion and encouragement and all of those good things listed in Philippians 2:1, we will start to care about people who are difficult to care for. We'll love people who are unlovely. We'll want to help people who don't like us and who have made life difficult for us. When you extend your hand to your "enemy"—whether a coworker who gets under your skin or a person who is openly hostile toward you—that's when you know that God's love is being made perfect in you, because that is what Jesus did. While we were His enemies, while we were still sinners, He died for us. (See Romans 5:8.)

Paul continues speaking about the importance of relationships in Philippians 2:2–4:

> *...then make my joy complete by being like-minded, having the same love, being one in spirit and of one mind. Do nothing out of selfish ambition or vain conceit. Rather, in humility value others above yourselves, not looking to your own interests but each of you to the interests of the others.*

Our loving, selfless relationships with others bring the unity that Jesus prayed for in John 17:21 when He asked God to make us one so that everyone would see how His followers love one another and would know that Jesus was who He said He was. (See also John

13:34–35.) Unity among believers points people to God and builds up the body of Christ. Once more, being in deep relationship with like-minded believers gives us support and encouragement. Knowing that there are people we can call in the middle of the night if something extraordinary—good or bad—happens is such a gift!

So, strong relationships bring us closer to God and give us security and support. They also influence our actions. When you look back on your life to the times when you were heading down a bad path, note who was influencing you at that point, who was speaking into your life. It probably wasn't a church community.

We love the idea of self-sufficiency and being able to be in control of outcomes in our lives. We don't want to depend on others, but that's exactly what God calls us to do. There is power in a holy relationship between kindred spirits. There is power in having people in your life who can come alongside you when you're slipping or struggling—people who will pray with you, weep with you, do life with you until you're back on your feet. This type of relationship is a glimpse of what God wants to have with us, and His making it possible for us to experience it with other believers shows His incredible love toward us.

PERFECT PRAISE

The best way to be in holy relationship with others is to chase after the mindset of Christ. Yet one tricky thing to navigate when it comes to taking on Christ's mindset is the fact that we all have a need to be exalted and praised. We were created in God's image, and, with that, we were given a natural desire to be lifted up. But, taking advantage of this God-given desire, Satan influences us to think we can handle God's job and that we should receive the same type of praise He receives. This is a distortion of the first commandment that Jesus expressed in Mark 12:30: *"Love the Lord your God with all your heart and with all your soul and with all your mind and with all your strength."* When we try to act in the place of God, we experience all sorts of anxiety and stressors if we aren't exalted in the way that we think we deserve to be. When we feel anxious over not receiving recognition for a job we did or over being slighted in some way, we can acknowledge to God how we feel and use that anxiety to cause us to return to His original design for us.

While we seek to be lifted up by other people, it is God who desires to exalt us! As we humble ourselves, He lifts us up, and, in doing this, He takes care of our anxiety (see 1 Peter 5:6–7), and He praises us for our humility.

While we are called to humble ourselves (see James 4:10; 1 Peter 5:6), humility is something that only God can work in us (see, for example, Daniel 4:37; James 3:13), and any success we have is through Him as well. He humbles us and then exalts us, and He does both of these things in the purest, most right way.

Humility is a very interesting thing. We can't be humble on our own. When we try, we either become prideful (the opposite of what we are trying to be) or depressed because we think humility means becoming a doormat for everyone to walk on. Perhaps our favorite definition of humility we've seen is this one: "Humility is not thinking less of yourself; it is just thinking of yourself less."[37] John the Baptist said, *"He* [Christ] *must become greater; I must become less"* (John 3:30).

When somebody compliments you or says something positive about you, do you always think of it as something random? Or might it be something that the Lord has planted in that person to say to you in order to build you up and, in turn, glorify the Father? (See Matthew 5:16.)

We might receive praise from others, but when we are close to Jesus, we know that only He is worthy of praise. We are broken vessels, but God works through us, and it's through this work that His name is lifted up.

---

37. This quote has often been attributed to C. S. Lewis, although he did not use these words. The idea may have come from Lewis's book *Mere Christianity*, book 3, chapter 8, where he discusses the nature of true humility using similar ideas. Whatever the origin of the quote, the concept it expresses is one that we (James and Ronnie) find very helpful as an encapsulation of the true meaning of humility.

There is something incredible about experiencing God in this way. Following Him and then seeing Him move in our lives is awe-inspiring and uplifting. But when we don't experience this relationship with God, we look elsewhere to be uplifted. We seek the praise of other people, and we end up becoming depressed because their words and their praise are not complete. Or we seek admiration in the workplace and come up short and with a head full of anxiety because things at work don't always go well; they're not always uplifting.

But when we depend on God to fill us up, we can expect to be complete.

PRACTICE AND EFFORT

Coming to a place where we trust and rely on God to give us what we need in our relationships requires practice and effort—and an intentional use of the algorithm can help with this.

Jesus was a realist. He acknowledged that each day brought struggle, and He advised us to not worry about the future—because there is enough for us to work through today! Jesus's strategy for getting through today was to live in God's kingdom. (See Matthew 6:33–34.)

When we live in our own kingdoms, we're responsible for everything. It's on us to make sure that things go the way we want them to and, more importantly, that needs are met and everyone is happy. It's an impossible task! This is why Jesus invites us to live in His kingdom, where all we have to do is trust that He will take care of us. Yes, there is hardship in life, but we don't need to be anxious about fixing it because Jesus is already at work.

The Chosen is a television program that depicts the lives of Jesus and His disciples. It brings the New Testament to life. We (James and Ronnie) love how the show portrays Jesus's humanity. In one of the early episodes, Jesus was new to His ministry, and, for the first time, He spent all day ministering to and healing people. When He got back to His tent, He collapsed on His bed because He was so drained of energy.

This is a side of Jesus that we don't often think about—the human side that had limits and felt fatigue, hunger, and pain. He lived in a human body just like we do. The difference between Jesus and us, however, is how He fully allowed the Holy Spirit to work through Him.

When you get inside Jesus's life, you find a Man of incredible peace. He truly set His mind on things above (see Colossians 3:2) and lived this out in a way that changed the world forever. He was all about the kingdom of God.

So, as you seek to follow Jesus's example, keep thinking about your mindset. Are you focused on the kingdom that you're trying to build with your career or aspirations or comfort? Is your motivation for wrangling your anxiety simply so that you can make life easier on yourself? Or are you focused on God's kingdom? Remember the growth mindset—God is working in you and through you for His glory and your good. You are not there yet, but He is moving you toward becoming all that He has in mind for you to be, and He wants you to step into this new life with confidence and joy.

Colossians 3 is such a powerful chapter about living out the Christian life in practical ways. It talks about the kingdoms of this world, which come with anger, rage, malice, slander, lying, and filthy language. It goes on to say that, in contrast, the kingdom of God comes with compassion, kindness, humility, gentleness, patience, forgiveness, love, and unity. And, it states that, as we live life in the kingdom of God, the peace of Christ will rule in our hearts. (See Colossians 3:8–15.) What a great promise!

We might have to live in a world full of human kingdoms, but we don't have to fit in with them. We don't have to participate in mindsets that are emotionally and spiritual harmful to us and others. We can choose a higher perspective that brings us peace and soundness of mind, and that's not just the Bible talking—as we have seen, science has also demonstrated it.

What does it mean to *choose* a higher mindset? There are many things that we understand and believe but don't act on. We may go to the doctor and discover that we are overweight, and we *know* we need to lose some pounds for our health and happiness, yet we return home and go back to our regular routines. We may find a leak in the attic, but instead of patching it right away, we place a bucket underneath it and hope for the best. Or we may realize that we don't always speak kindly to our children or spouse. Instead of immediately working on improving our communication, we let it slide. There are many things like these and more—all good things to do!—that we cognitively understand but don't put into practice. We have to make a specific commitment to changing our approach to them.

In Philippians, Paul says that we can make plans all we want, but we also have to put in the work. We have to put in effort. And this doesn't just mean putting in the effort to root out the things that are causing us trouble. It means putting in the effort to reshape our thoughts, to improve our lives, and to create more beauty in them.

CHOOSING YOUR MINDSET

So much of choosing your mindset comes down to making a decision and sticking to it. But, more importantly, if you ask, God is able to help you to do this by His Spirit. When you feel yourself being pulled away from a kingdom mindset, you can rely on the Spirit to bring you back to center.

The world will tell you that you need to work harder, be more talented, look prettier, and so forth, but the Spirit's main message for you is simple: He offers a life of peace. Any time you feel confused or unloved, that is not from God. The Holy Spirit does not bring confusion. If you keep seeking Him, He will either bring clarity to your situation or ask you to continue to trust Him as He works out His perfect will in your life. *"For we live by believing and not by seeing"* (2 Corinthians 5:7 NLT). And, remember, any time you feel inferior or down on yourself, that is not of the Spirit. Any time you feel weak or threatened or inadequate, that is not of the Spirit. Whenever you feel any of these things, run to God, and He will make you strong. He will make you whole. He will fill in the gaps in your life that the world can't help but point out to you. When you are distressed in this way, using the Anxiety Algorithm will help you to run to Him.

God will enable you to set your mind on things above if you ask and abide in Him. All you have to do is take two steps back from that spiraling mindset and invite the Spirit to take control. Rest in His peace. Relinquish those burdens that the world is piling on you.

In addition to calling upon the Spirit, you can practice taking Scripture to heart. Remember, Jesus defeated Satan's temptations by quoting Scripture. That's all He did! Ask God to reveal what He says about you through His Word—you might be surprised.

As we have previously emphasized, following these practices will require lots of intentionality at first. But, over time, this posture and mindset will be reflexive. It will be your natural state of being!

I want to remind you of one thing that I (Ronnie) have found about trusting God with hardship: He seems to take all of the bad, all of the difficulty, all of the suffering, and box it up; then He transforms it into something amazing. I've seen Him do this so many times that, now, when I face hardship, I can't wait to see what He's going to do with it! I can't wait for the beautiful end result. Don't get me wrong: it's not that I want hardship to happen to me or to anyone else, but hardship is a part of life. The difference is that, when hardship occurs, my mindset has been renewed. Instead of asking God why He would let such a thing happen, I ask Him to please not let me miss what He has for me in that hardship.

If you're looking for an example of God doing the same thing in someone else's life, remember that you need look no further than the life of Jesus. He was called to the cross—something that He struggled with so much. He sweat and bled as He prayed, asking for there to be another way. But God took the hardship, the pain—all of Jesus's suffering—and brought tremendous victory out of it. Jesus rose from the grave and saved humanity from eternal death. *"For the joy set before him he endured the cross"* (Hebrews 12:2).

Jesus understands the struggle involved in choosing to "delight in hardship" (see 2 Corinthians 12:10) because He lived it. He experienced it. And He shows us that when our minds are fixed on the right things, we have an opportunity to connect with God and experience the joy that comes from His presence.

We can practice choosing a kingdom mindset by following God every day. There is so much we can learn from Jesus if we just walk with Him. Satan wants you to believe that God doesn't have your best interests in mind—that His way will be undesirable and unfair. Satan wants you to believe that you can't trust God for the abundant life He promises. (See John 10:10 ESV, KJV.) He wants you to strive for God's favor and try to earn His blessing. But Jesus has already done everything necessary for you to have the abundant life He promised. This reality is affirmed in 2 Peter 1:3–4, Romans 5:1–2, and Ephesians 1:3. We need to keep this truth in mind: if we are in Christ, we have it all. How's that for a mindset shift?

WE REPRESENT THE KINGDOM

Having a kingdom mindset not only helps us to align our perspectives with Jesus's and to live life in Him, but it also enables us to be God's representatives to others.

> *Do everything without grumbling or arguing, so that you may become blameless and pure, "children of God without fault in a warped and crooked generation." Then you will shine among them like stars in the sky as you hold firmly to the word of life.*
> (Philippians 2:14–16)

This world is going to cause you to want to grumble and argue because there are people in it, and people are messy. The church is made up of a bunch of sinners, and we don't get things right much of the time. Really, if you read the Bible from cover to cover, you will discover that it is a continuous story of people who struggled to get it right, and who got it wrong a lot of times. From the very beginning, God knew there was only one solution: the Man Jesus.

We in the church often cause more problems than we solve, and we can make following Jesus look pretty unappealing. That's why we need to adopt a kingdom mindset—so that even our relationships within the church can be transformed for God's glory, drawing others closer to Him.

If you've ever been out in the open countryside on a dark night, you've likely been mesmerized by how many stars you can see and how they look. They twinkle and shine and put on an awe-inducing show. We both (James and Ronnie) live out in the country in the middle of the woods. Many times, on a clear, moonless night, we can even see the Milky Way, and it is absolutely spectacular. Imagine if every single one of us Jesus followers were to shine just like that in this dark world. Imagine if we were to capture the attention of those around us, making them wonder how we were able to shine so brightly.

This world is dark. But as we live with our minds fixed on God's kingdom, we're able to enjoy life here on earth. The early church exemplified this. They lived in a Roman-occupied world, and the Roman world didn't leave much room for Christianity. In fact, at times, it did everything it could to destroy it. But those in the early church experienced such joy from their relationships with Jesus and each other that, when they went out and talked about the good news of Jesus Christ, God was glorified, people were drawn in, the name of Jesus spread, and the church grew!

People wanted to know why these oppressed Jesus followers were happier than everyone around them—they just had to see what this new Way was all about. The believers in the early church were stars shining in the darkness.

WHEN TO INTERVENE

Having the right mindset is so important because anxious thoughts come from a flesh-based mentality. Developing a kingdom mindset can keep us on course and slowly refine us into being kingdom-focused. But, sometimes, often at a moment's notice, we need to take action in a way that goes beyond the gradual process of working on our mindset. We need to intervene in life, and this is not an easy thing.

Paul understood this when he sent Epaphroditus home to Philippi. (See Philippians 2:25–30.) We talked about aspects of this story in earlier chapters. Paul was experiencing anxiety and stress because his close coworker Epaphroditus had been gravely sick, and Epaphroditus's fellow church members in Philippi had heard about his illness and were worried about him. So, Paul needed to do something about it. The Spirit revealed to him that an intervention was *necessary*, that sending Epaphroditus home was the right thing to do to restabilize both Paul's mission and the church in Philippi. And so Paul made the difficult decision to take action, even though it meant being separated from his dear friend and reliable coworker in the gospel.

We can have the right mindset and know the right things and have the Spirit, but if we lack action when it counts, it can all be for nothing. This is what we mean by the importance of taking intervention when needed.

As we expressed above, one of the worst things we can do is to sit on something that we know we're supposed to do. I (Ronnie) am great at this! I have notebooks filled with plans and aspirations and projects that would really make a difference, but there hasn't been any movement toward them on my part. It's like when we show up at church on Sunday morning and get inspired by the message but then don't do the hard work of changing, growing, surrendering to God, and turning our lives around. We don't just need inspiration—we need transformation!

Sometimes it's hard to imagine a life in which you can actually get ahead of your stress and anxiety, but it's possible. The key is to take two steps back as soon as you feel the stress and anxiety coming on. The sooner you can zoom out and see the big picture, the more likely you are to prevent a mental and emotional spiral. And sometimes seeing that big picture helps you to take a needed act of intervention.

Let's say you're someone who struggles with social anxiety, and you're late for church. You've got young kids, and getting both yourself and them ready that morning has been hard, so you're already stressed out. The fact that you're late for church is creating some anxious thoughts. Ideally, you'd stop right there, take two steps back, and run through the algorithm until you felt refocused and more at peace. But let's say you allow the thoughts to continue, and they build. You think about a spotlight being on you when you walk in late. You worry over not being able to find a seat. You worry over what others will think and what they'll say.

At this point, you have a decision to make: you can stay home, or you can push through the anxiety and go to church and face your stress. If you go to church, you're choosing to intervene by taking immediate action to counteract your anxiety. You might have some uncomfortable interactions, but, overall, you'll likely feel pretty good about yourself for having done the hard thing. If you stay home, your anxious thoughts might subside—or they might just get worse. You might experience shame or even embarrassment over your decision. You might start to worry about friends asking you where you were.

Taking action and intervening can many times stop an anxiety spiral—but intervention is hard! It's much easier to give in to your fears and stressors and try to protect yourself from them, only to reap the consequences later when your mind refuses to let go of the very fears and worries that you're trying to protect yourself from.

The earlier we can intervene in this thought process, the better. The sooner we can remind ourselves, "Jesus will love me whether I'm late or on time," the sooner we can implement deep breathing, and the sooner we can take two steps back, the better.

Anxiety is like having someone constantly tug at your sleeve. Most of the time, it doesn't bother you too much. You're able to go through life and think about other things. But when you are faced with stress or fear or worry, suddenly that tugging becomes unbearable, and the next thing you know, you're snapping over something small because you've been living with that constant annoyance, that constant reminder, that things could go bad at any moment.

If you never address that tugging, you'll never experience the freedom and clarity God has for you. The problem that causes the tugging might not fully go away, but you can change your mindset in a way that frees you from being pulled down by your burden.

At first, you might find that you have to do a lot of intervening in your life. You may find that your habits and mindsets are so far off track that you need to take what might feel like drastic measures to work toward wellness. Don't let this discourage you. It is much better to do the hard work of intervention than to continue living a life of anxiety with an unawareness of God's presence.

STAGES OF CHANGE

Many rehab groups focus on the five stages of change. While these stages are especially relevant for those dealing with addiction, we (James and Ronnie) have found them to be helpful for nearly any mental difficulty that people are trying to overcome. In an article published online by the National Institutes of Health, the authors give a more complete overview of each stage, which we have briefly summarized below:

Stage 1: Precontemplation. This is the period of time before you know that you need to change.

Stage 2: Contemplation. This is when you start to realize that you might need to change, or that there's an issue that needs to be dealt with.

Stage 3: Preparation. This is when you aren't taking much action, but you're processing and thinking about your problem. You're trying to develop a plan and find helpful resources.

Stage 4: Action. This is when you finally take steps of change.

Stage 5: Maintenance (habit created). This is when you begin to turn your action into a new habit that becomes the new normal for you.[38]

---

38. Nahrain Raihan and Mark Cogburn, "Stages of Change Theory," National Institute of Health, March 6, 2023, National Library of Medicine, https://www.ncbi.nlm.nih.gov/books/NBK556005/.

The first thing about these stages that should jump out at you is that when you choose to take action, you are already at stage 4 (although, as the article points out, the preparation stage is an essential preliminary step). How encouraging is that?

If we use the goal of weight loss as an example of this process, then it typically looks like this: You're living life, not thinking too much about your weight (stage 1), but then you visit the doctor or step on the scale or find that your clothes don't fit the way they used to, and you realize you have a problem (stage 2). You research diets and exercise programs to find something that works for your goals and lifestyle (stage 3). You begin to change your eating habits and to move your body more, and you see some results (stage 4). You then implement this diet and exercise program into your life moving forward, because you don't want to go back to who you were before. You want this change to last (stage 5). It's in stage 5 that you finally begin to experience this new lifestyle in a reflexive way. In each of the previous stages, you had to plan and be intentional about each step and choice, but, over time, as your new diet becomes a habit, it's reflexive. The things you used to do that got you to a point of being overweight do not have the appeal that they once did!

One way to start this process is to change your mindset about the way that you want to feel. This is what we (James and Ronnie) describe as the "stress-can-be-enhancing mindset," a concept discussed by Dr. Alia Crum.[39] This means to accept some of the discomfort (stress) of change in order to accomplish your purpose. For example, in changing your mindset about weight loss, you begin by making it your goal to experience what it feels like to get in shape (even with the accompanying tiredness) rather than having a goal of losing weight. In other words, when your goal is in the effort and not in a number, you can celebrate each day. It doesn't matter what the scale says. What matters is what you accomplished that day to help you move toward wellness.

This change in mindset may seem like a small thing, but it can make a huge difference. Instead of aiming to lose weight, you shift

---

39. Crum, "Science of Mindsets for Health and Performance, 45:00.

your focus to feeling more energetic and active. You'll go from wanting to have a full stomach to embracing the hunger you may feel at times. You'll go from wanting to sit around comfortably to embracing the discomfort and fatigue of movement and exercise. Instead of viewing tired muscles as a bad thing, you'll begin to see them as a sign that you're doing something right! Experiencing fatigue and pain and sweat means that you are changing.

In time, you will go from someone who avoids pain and discomfort, who relies too much on food for happiness, to someone who embraces tired muscles and who eats for fuel. You will be a changed person because you will have a changed mindset.

Improving one's physical health, losing weight, building muscles—these are easy examples because they are common struggles. But the same stress-can-be-enhancing mindset that can be used for physical health can also be used for mental health.

The key is this: the clearer your plan, the easier it will be to implement, and the greater chance it will have at success. Refer to your anxiety algorithm and thought record often to help you develop and maintain your plan.

HARD BUT WORTH IT

The more you implement daily wellness practices and rightfully address issues with intervention, the more life-changing results you will see. The peace you will feel, the joy you will experience, the hope you will have for a life lived with your Lord—those feelings will be indescribable.

But it all starts with the hard work. It takes time to make new habits and crush old ones. Yet don't forget that Jesus is with you, offering you strength, support, love, patience, and, of course, forgiveness for every misstep along the way.

20

DISCOVERING TRUE JOY

Philippians 3 is all about joy. Right in the first verse, Paul says, *"Further, my brothers and sisters, rejoice in the Lord! It is no trouble for me to write the same things to you again, and it is a safeguard for you."*

Joy is part of our Christian faith, and, according to Paul, joy is found in Christ and in relationships with other people. However, if you've struggled with anxiety, joy might seem distant. It might seem like something other people have, not you. Sure, you may feel happy every once in a while, and there might be parts of your life that you are thankful for. But joy? A life of joy does not go hand in hand with a life of anxiety. Replacing your anxiety with peace will bring the joy that God promises. But how, exactly, can you do that? In Philippians, Paul explains that proper perspectives, and their resulting actions, can change our lives in a way that brings true joy.

JOY KEEPS US SAFE

The reason joy is so important is explained in Philippians 3:1: *"it is a safeguard."* Joy guards us and keeps us safe. Furthermore, it is a place of habit. We return to the things that bring us joy, so if our joy comes from Jesus, then that is where we'll put our time and attention. Jesus is the water that doesn't run dry (see John 4:14; 6:35; 7:37–38), and so, while most things of this world can bring temporary joy, He brings a fullness of joy that transforms lives. This is because the joy found in Jesus comes from within us, where His Spirit resides. It's not based on circumstances or other people. It's inside us whether we're facing hardship or experiencing goodness.

But, too often, our joy gets tangled up in the wrong things. According to Paul, people and things can quickly steal our joy.

"WHATEVER WERE GAINS TO ME..."

In Philippians 3, the first warning Paul gives regarding joy is about other people. Of all of the things that can affect our joy and pull us away from Jesus, *people* is number one. And the people who threaten our joy the most are those who do not have their eyes on Jesus. They give bad advice and encourage bad behavior that leads to poor consequences, and they pull us further and further away from Him.

In my (Ronnie's) pediatric practice, I met regularly with teenagers who were dealing with some bad consequences. When I would walk them back to figure out how it all started, almost every time, it would come down to what they called FOMO: fear of missing out.

They were worried that if they didn't go along with things that their friends were doing, they would be forgotten about, left behind, or seen as insignificant. They were convinced that joy and fulfillment would be found in following the advice and actions of others, and so they would attach themselves to people who came across as strong, popular, successful, and charismatic. But, so often, those people led them into darkness.

It's easy to shake our heads at their ignorance, but this very thing happens to us adults too. We put our confidence in people and things, much as teenagers do. We place our trust and expectations in our health insurance, our standard of living, our retirement funds, our church leaders, our employers or employees, our businesses, our politicians, our appearance, and our social clout. Relying on some of these things isn't always bad, but it can become bad when an obsession about them takes over. When we're always checking our stock investments, or when we spend hours and hours at the gym every single day, we might be trusting in people and things more than in Christ. Hopefully, we can trust our church community, but what happens when we begin to exalt one of the leaders, or when we try to gain more power there? Or what happens when our career becomes our primary focus or our identity?

One way to know if you're clinging to something too tightly is to watch what happens when things go badly in relation to it. What happens to you when the stock market drops, one of your employees walks out, business is down, you don't get the promotion you were hoping for, your political party loses an election, or your spouse doesn't support you in the way you had hoped? How do you handle it? If anxiety or anger or panic wells up within you, then you know you're trying to find your identity and your joy in that thing and not in Christ.

Paul understood this. As he expressed in the passage below, he was of the tribe of Benjamin and a zealous Pharisee who persecuted the church and sought righteousness based on the law. In other words, Paul had put a lot of stock in who he was and what he believed, and, as a result, he had been at the top of the Jewish social hierarchy of the time. A chief priest ranking had likely been in his future, and yet all of that no longer mattered to him. He had come face-to-face with God's "*whatever*":

In Philippians 3:4–9, Paul writes:

> *If someone else thinks they have reasons to put confidence in the flesh, I have more: circumcised on the eighth day, of the people of Israel, of the tribe of Benjamin, a Hebrew of Hebrews; in regard to the law, a Pharisee; as for zeal, persecuting the church; as for righteousness based on the law, faultless. But* **whatever** *were*

gains to me I now consider loss for the sake of Christ. What is more, I consider everything a loss because of the surpassing worth of knowing Christ Jesus my Lord, for whose sake I have lost all things. I consider them garbage, that I may gain Christ and be found in him, not having a righteousness of my own that comes from the law, but that which is through faith in Christ.

What "gains" do you fear losing? And what does that fear do for your anxiety?

When my children were young, I (Ronnie) took them to see where I grew up. As soon as we pulled off the road, my daughter Emily (who was twelve at the time) said, "I don't know if you're aware of this, Dad, but I think you grew up in poverty."

I'd never thought of it that way, but as I looked at my childhood home through her eyes, I saw a simple home with walls that were the same on the outside as they were on the inside—no insulation or drywall. When it got cold, we'd had to huddle by the heater to stay warm.

Still, I had lacked nothing. My parents had provided me with what I needed, and I was able to attend Mississippi State and then medical school. Because of this, I had never truly considered the economic nature of my upbringing, but Emily was right. After medical school, I found myself in a different economic circle, and, at some point along the way, someone gave me a Montblanc pen as a gift. These are very nice, very expensive pens, and I treasured that gift and kept it with me, thinking that I would never let it go. It symbolized that I had made it as a doctor.

And then I lost the pen.

I went through the house, looking inside every box, every possible hiding spot. I moped around and couldn't stop talking about the pen, wondering where it was. And then, one day, I opened a desk drawer, and there it was.

The very next week, I was teaching Sunday school, and I asked the group what they feared losing the most. What material thing were they holding on to? What did they cherish more than their relationship with God?

It's amazing how oblivious I can be, because the pen didn't even cross my mind until the words were out of my mouth. It's as if God were standing before me shining a big spotlight on my sin. Right there, I took the pen out of my pocket and showed it to the class. That insignificant possession had a grip on me, and the thought of losing it again made me anxious.

That's how you know you're putting your confidence in something other than the joy and peace that God has for you. There's nothing wrong with enjoying a pen—but the way I held on to and uplifted that pen was sinful!

A similar thing happened to me with iPhones. In the past, I would research the new models for three or four months before they hit the shelves. I knew all of the bells and whistles. I knew how the phones compared to older models, and I couldn't wait to get my hands on one.

What did that obsession get me? Did it bring peace? Joy? Fulfillment? No, it brought a temporary high and a distraction from the things in life that really mattered. Today, I have a box of old iPhones collecting dust in the garage—phones I paid top dollar for as soon as they hit retail!

So, when I think about the "gains" of this world, I think about material possessions, social status, economic status, relational clout—all things that will come and go. But God's love and the peace He offers are constant. They have never changed. They have been there for me through great times and bad times, too. They have seen me through, and they have done a whole lot more for me than any pen or iPhone ever did.

What is your "whatever" when it comes to worldly gains? And how much of a grip does it have on your anxiety? How is it keeping you stuck in your current pattern, away from joy, away from peace, away from the life God has for you?

OUR SOURCE OF RIGHTEOUSNESS

Just as we can hold tightly to the wrong things, we can also depend on the wrong things to help us achieve righteousness.

Righteousness is the state of being right with God. But how can something like that be determined? How can we know that we are right, or not right, with the Lord?

Righteousness comes from God on the basis of our faith in Christ, but most of us try to point to external things to prove that we are, in fact, right with God. We may read our Bible every day, pray regularly, and tithe our income. We may attend church every week. We may lead a church group and mentor other believers. None of these things is bad. In fact, they are very beneficial for helping us and others grow in our Christian faith. But they are works, and when we are depending upon our works to achieve righteous standing with God, we're going to live very anxious lives.

There is only one act of righteousness that God accepts, and that is what His Son did on the cross. When we live as though our salvation depends more on what we do than on what Christ has already accomplished, we are going to struggle. We're going to be anxious and depressed because we're going to come up short. But when we realize that our righteousness before God is based totally on what Jesus has done for us, things change. Yes, we are still affected by hardship and pain, but, in those moments, we more readily go back to the cross, acknowledging that we are powerless to help and save ourselves, and trusting in Jesus to deliver us.

You will find that the algorithm helps with this. It will bring you back to the cross when your mind is racing with anxious thoughts that pull you away from recognizing that Jesus paid it all.

I (Ronnie) love my wife, and if she tells me to do something, I do it—not because I'm trying to prove my love for her or earn her favor, but because I trust her. I trust that she's looking out for me and that her requests are for my own good and for the good of our family. This is the type of trust relationship that God wants to have with us, where we abide in His love and rest in the assurance that He does and always will look after us.

You might let go of Jesus, but He's not going to let go of you. You might let go of His hand, but He's got a firm grip on your arm, and there's nothing you can do to change that. He desires a relationship that is based on His love for you, and He takes hold of you because He wants to lead you into your best. He wants you to be the best spouse, the best parent, the best teacher, the best coach, the best employee—and He will see you through!

When I (Ronnie) began speaking at schools to teach educators about the treatment of children with school problems, there were times when people would pack out a gymnasium just to listen to me share. There would be hundreds of people crammed on the bleachers, waiting to hear what I had to say. My nerves got hold of me, and I developed some serious GI issues. I began to take medicine and to structure my day around those issues so that they wouldn't be a problem when I spoke. Then I realized that it was God who had brought me to this place and blessed my speaking ministry. He wanted me in those packed gymnasiums, and He was responsible for the results, not me. I could prepare and study and pray, but everything depended on Him—even my health and nerves.

Immediately, my anxiety settled, and my GI issues cleared up.

When you realize that God is responsible for what He wants to accomplish through you, you can let go of the things that get in your way. This clears the way for you to experience joy in Christ. When you live in the reality that God loves you and wants what's best for you, then being in right relationship with Him is all that matters, and from that springs joy.

SETTING BOUNDARIES

Christians can struggle with setting appropriate boundaries in life because we tend to believe that following Jesus means we always help and serve and give sacrificially, no matter what. We believe it's rude and even sinful to say no when people come to us with needs or requests. But when our lives are full of responsibilities and relationships that take and take from us, and we don't have boundaries set in place to ensure that we remain healthy and centered on the things that are most important, we can become overextended and miserable. We can end up worshipping at the altar of service and sacrifice rather than worshipping the King. This will inevitably affect our joy. We will become bitter and exhausted, and the skills and talents that we once used so gladly for the kingdom will become joyless obligations.

Boundaries give us freedom. They make it clear when it's okay to say no to an opportunity or to a request to help meet a certain need. The opportunity might be good and worthy, or the need might be legitimate. But it might not be the right thing for us to be involved in at that time—and boundaries help us to determine that. Remember, God doesn't *need* us to accomplish His work. He enjoys partnering with us, but we are not solely responsible for spreading His kingdom on earth. We have a role to play in what He's doing, but that role isn't always a leading one.

If you're someone who struggles with guilt when saying no, then you need to pray through that and seek the Lord's help. By "pray through," I mean commit to praying about this issue and meditating on what is true, right, noble, and so forth in regard to it until you are able to release the feelings of guilt and obligation and set healthy boundaries on your time and commitments. Jesus Himself knew when it was time for Him to get away and rest. He knew when to close down His ministry for the day and spend time with His friends. Over thirty times in the book of Luke, we read that Jesus sought out time alone with God. He modeled what it means to set healthy boundaries.

Some years ago, my wife, Anne, and I (Ronnie) volunteered to go on church youth group trips. At that time, we couldn't afford vacations, and the youth group was always glad to have a doctor help chaperone their trips, so we'd go along and have some great experiences with our kids. But there was one particular trip that felt different to me. I felt like I wasn't supposed to go on it. I prayed about it and talked to Anne, and she felt like she wasn't supposed to go either. Even though it was hard to let the church know we wouldn't be accompanying the group this time, we stood firm in our decision because we just did not have a peace about going.

Someone else volunteered to help chaperone the trip, and, to this day, that person will tell you that the trip was a big turning point in their life. It solidified some things that God was working on within them.

Seeing the need, I could have felt pressure to go on the trip. But if I had ignored God's voice telling me to sit this one out, that other believer wouldn't have had the experience they did. Sometimes saying no isn't a good thing—it's the best thing.

I remember one day when our children were still very young, and I came home to find Anne—who doesn't usually get upset—calm but noticeably bothered. "I need to tell you something. I don't know how you're going to take it," she said, "but you're neglecting your family, and I'm not talking about your work."

Those were hard words to hear. I was running a medical practice in addition to being a husband and father. On top of that, I was *the* guy whom everyone seemed to rely on at church. I loved serving in that way, and I remember wondering how it could possibly be wrong to give so much of my time to the church! I felt that the congregation could not survive without my presence on every committee. The people *needed* me to be at every meeting and help make all the decisions.

But I decided to take two steps back to get a different perspective, and God revealed to me that Anne was right. At that moment, I had a decision to make. I could keep doing things my way, or I could intervene in my life and take big, scary steps toward change. I chose intervention. The next day, I stepped down from all five committees I was on at church. (There are some things we can [and should] immediately remove from our schedule, and other things we may need to gradually step back from, depending on the situation. Ultimately, we must prayerfully reach a point of healthy balance in our responsibilities.) To my disappointment, my church did just fine without me; and, in some ways, it got better.

This was a powerful lesson, showing me how I had allowed my desire to serve the Lord to infringe upon my calling as a husband and father. I had been allowing my pride to direct my steps, not my humility, and that's when I got off base.

Those were painful experiences, but they were necessary. Today, I automatically say no to an opportunity unless it has been made clear to me that God is in it. I think that, in return, I have been less neglectful of my family *and* have been doing more of what God really wants me to do instead of spending time on small things that I thought would bring me prestige or admiration or bonus points. And, ultimately, I've found so much more joy. My outlook on life is at peace. Instead of running around, thinking that I need to solve all the problems around me and serve until I've run myself ragged, I now operate out of joyful energy, and every one of my acts of service to the Lord is done in abundance and with a joyful heart. It has been good for me and good for those I care for deeply.

PRESSING ON

Brothers and sisters, I do not consider myself yet to have taken hold of it. But one thing I do: Forgetting what is behind and straining toward what is ahead, I press on toward the goal to win the prize for which God has called me heavenward in Christ Jesus. (Philippians 3:13–14)

This passage shows that Paul came across resistance in his journey with God. He was doing what he could to press in and push forward to the goal of knowing and being known by Jesus. He left his past behind him while he focused on abiding in Christ.

It's easy to let our past steal our joy. It's easy to wallow in the should-have-beens or to feel shame and regret for things that we have done. We learn from our past, yes, but we shouldn't live there. If you struggle with doing that, if the past is an anchor that is keeping you from being all that God wants you to be, then you need to pray about those chains.

It's time we viewed hardship and stressors as opportunities for God to make us stronger and more like Him. He allows these things to help us change our mindset and grow, and to help us shift from being intentional to being reflexive. It's when we get emotional about the stressors in our lives that we begin to crumble, so that's why it's important to take two steps back when conflict or stress first hits. It's going to be tempting to take two steps forward and to get back in the thick of it, but if we do that, we will hinder God from working.

It isn't our job to figure everything out. But we can ask God to help us see a situation through His eyes. When we can see the role we played in a spiraling relationship or an anxiety-producing scenario, we begin to see more clearly. And, by abiding in Christ, we find that instead of bringing us down, those past mistakes can bring praise to our lips as God reveals to us areas in which we can grow and change. He delivers us—even those of us who have been following Him for years!

When you start to ask God to give you His eyes, you'll be amazed. Your emotions will calm, and you'll become less defensive. The conflict you face will take a back seat to the care and love you have for the people involved—people you may previously have struggled to get along with. You'll begin to make things right; you'll begin to apologize. Then, watch God use that. Just like Joseph did in the Old Testament, watch God bring good out of a bad situation.

Years ago, in our backyard, I (James) had a little above-ground fire pit that I would light so that I could burn leaves and sticks to clean up the yard. My boys loved to come out there and sit around the fire, throwing pine cones and twigs into it. It was usually a great time.

However, one day, I was across the yard when I looked over to check on the boys at the fire pit, and they were having an argument. My six-year-old was trying to tip my four-year-old's chair into the fire! Instantly, I was in a rage and charged over to them.

But the fire pit was fifteen steps away from me. And, in those fifteen steps, I was able to think about the situation. My six-year-old wasn't actually trying to dump my four-year-old into the fire. He was just trying to scare him. So, during the time it took me to reach the boys, I was able to realize that it would do no good if I went in there with the intent to bring punishment. If I charged in with anger and fury, nothing would be accomplished. By the time I got there, I was calm and thinking clearly. I rescued my four-year-old, then pulled my six-year-old aside and had a teaching moment with him instead of a moment of rage that I would have forever regretted.

When we're in the moment of stress or anxiety, God wants us to take the extra time to see things clearly from His perspective. The more we do this, the easier it gets. My emotions got me running toward the fire, but God's presence showed me the right way to handle the situation.

I (Ronnie) would use my private bathroom at my medical practice to take two steps back when needed. If I was about to see a patient who was difficult, if I had handled something badly, or if I was feeling the stress of a situation, I would go in there and pray. In that bathroom, my wife had hung a framed list of the fruit of the Spirit, with ten little handprints from my ten grandchildren. What a powerful reminder that was! It was not just about my representing Jesus. It was about my being an example to my family. I can't explain the joy that came as a result of using that space in that way. I was able to stay centered and have fewer regrets over the course of my day. And I was able to more keenly feel the presence of God as I visited patient after patient. What joy that brought!

The Anxiety Algorithm will help you to capture the same joy as it centers you in Christ in the midst of the chaos of life. And a life of joy is a life of clarity, righteousness, and peace with God.

◇ ◇ ◇

WELLNESS EXERCISE: ENGAGE IN SPIRITUAL PRACTICES

Not that I have already obtained all this, or have already arrived at my goal, but I press on to take hold of that for which Christ Jesus took hold of me. (Philippians 3:12)

How are you "pressing on" in your relationship with Jesus? Having spiritual wellness requires that we spend time with our Savior, Jesus Christ. Practices that assist us in doing this, such as Bible reading, Scripture memorization, and prayer, are known as spiritual disciplines.

When we are trying to exercise to get in better shape, we engage in disciplines or activities we know will help us achieve our goal. The same is true in our walk with Jesus. If we want to abide in Him (see John 15:5 ESV) so that we are in His will and producing spiritual fruit, we have to engage in those activities that help us to do so.

I (James) remember my pastor using an illustration one time during a sermon when trying to help people understand why we need to read the Bible, pray, memorize Scripture, and so forth. He said that if we didn't reach out to God in these ways, it would be like a bride and groom getting married but, after the ceremony, living in two different houses and never interacting. They would still be married, but they would not have a relationship with each other.

Similarly, you may make the decision to follow Jesus, but do you spend time with Him? One of our previous wellness exercises was about establishing a daily quiet time. Now, in this exercise, we encourage you to intentionally think through all of your various spiritual practices. Simply going to church a few times a month or even every week does not mean you have a relationship with Jesus. This is why we *must* read the Bible often, pray often, and memorize Scripture often. These practices help us to understand who God is and the nature of His purposes and ways. They enable us to express our love for Him and learn how to love other people. And they give God an opportunity to express His love and His thoughts toward us.

How many times per week do you read the Bible with the goal of getting to know God better?

How often do you pray? Do you pray only when you need something, or do you have an ongoing conversation with God throughout your day as though He were walking around with you?

Do you memorize Scripture so that the Holy Spirit can bring it to mind when you need to remember it?

Do you fellowship with other believers regularly and talk about what Jesus is doing in your life?

Do a self-examination and really think through whether you are engaging Jesus on a regular basis. The truth is that reading your Bible or praying, in itself, won't change you. It is Jesus who changes you through the power of His Spirit. But, again, starting each day by reading your Bible and praying does create opportunities for Him to speak to you and for you to learn more about who He is and who He has made you to be.

21

THE ALGORITHM AND PRAYER

The Anxiety Algorithm works because, having a relationship with Jesus, we can base our affirmations about what is true, noble, right, pure, lovely, admirable, excellent, and praiseworthy on the spiritual realities of our life in Him. However, as we have seen, for any relationship to be strong, the parties have to be able to communicate with each other; they have to talk to one another. That's what prayer is for.

The practice of prayer is an important part of our spiritual and emotional wellness. It is so important that John the Baptist taught his followers how to pray (see Luke 11:1), and Jesus taught His disciples great truths about prayer, including the manner in which we should go about praying and what elements we should include in prayer. (See, for example, Matthew 6:5–14.)

But there's one line from Jesus that trips many of us up to this day: *"Your Father knows what you need before you ask him"* (Matthew 6:8).

If God knows what we need, why ask? If He knows what we're thinking and feeling, then what's the point of telling Him what He already knows? This kind of thinking can lead to questions such as, "What's the purpose of running through the algorithm if Jesus already knows what I'm struggling with?"

This is just one of the many mental blocks we may experience when it comes to prayer. Some of us may also struggle with doubting that our prayers will actually result in movement from God. We may have become disappointed in prayers that have been left, in our opinion, unanswered. And some of us just don't make the time to talk with God.

Regardless of what we may have thought and felt about prayer in the past, if we want the algorithm to work, if we want God to move in our lives, then we need to get serious about praying. It's time for us to rethink how and why we pray.

TALKING WITH GOD

> *Rejoice in the Lord always. I will say it again: Rejoice! Let your gentleness be evident to all. The Lord is near. Do not be anxious about anything, but in every situation, by prayer and petition, with thanksgiving, present your requests to God. And the peace of God, which transcends all understanding, will guard your hearts and your minds in Christ Jesus.* (Philippians 4:4–7)

Parents often have a sixth sense for what their children need. Without their asking, a parent can tell when their child is tired, hungry, sad, or lonely. Regardless of the circumstances, there is something that lights up within a parent when they spend time with their child. And it's even better when the child is honest about what they need and what they're struggling with. It may not be new information—the parent might already know the stressors and issues that their child is facing—but talking with them about it takes it to the next level.

Much as we love talking with our children and friends, whether they are going through good times or bad, God enjoys talking to us at any time. Moreover, no relationship exists in a vacuum. If we are going to have a relationship with God, we simply have to talk to Him!

NAME ABOVE ALL NAMES

It's easy to see God as one-dimensional when He is actually multifaceted. He isn't merely a Friend, a Comforter, a King, or a Judge. He is *everything* good and right and just.

The Bible offers numerous names for God. We often see this pattern in the Scriptures: God moves, and then, in response to His movement, the people (or person) involved attribute to God a name that reflects what He did or how He worked. These names are incredibly powerful because they are true. They represent who God is and what He has done and is doing. And these are names through which we can honor Him with praise and call on Him in prayer.

Some of the names of God, along with some scriptural examples of their use, include the following:[40]

- *Elohim*: "God, Judge, Creator"; "the Sovereign, Mighty Creator" (See Genesis 1:1, 26.)
- *Jehovah Adonai*: "The Lord God"; "Jehovah Is the Lord"; "Master, Owner, or Lord" (See Genesis 15:2, 8; Judges 6:22.)
- *El Shaddai*: "God Almighty"; "God Is the All-Powerful One"; "The All-Sufficient One" (See Genesis 17:1; 28:3.)
- *Jehovah Jireh*: "The Lord Will Provide" (See Genesis 22:8; 13–15.)
- *Jehovah Rapha*: "The Lord Who Heals You"; "The Lord My Health" (See Exodus 15:26.)

---

40. The names of God and their definitions in this chapter are taken from these sources: "The Hebrew Names and Attributes of God," in the King James Version Easy Read Bible, KJVER™, © 2001, 2007, 2010, 2015, 2023 by Global Evangelism, Inc. Used by permission. All rights reserved; Marilyn Hickey, *The Names of God* (New Kensington, PA: Whitaker House, 2009). Used by permission; and "The Names of God in the Old Testament," Blue Letter Bible, https://www.blueletterbible.org/study/misc/name_god.cfm.

- *Jehovah Nissi*: "The Lord My Banner" (See Exodus 17:15.)
- *Jehovah M'Kaddesh*: "The Lord Who Sanctifies You" (See Exodus 31:13; Leviticus 20:7–8; Ezekiel 20:12.)
- *Jehovah Shalom*: "The Lord Is Peace"; "The Lord Is My Peace and Wholeness" (See Judges 6:23–24.)
- *Jehovah Sabaoth*: "The Lord of Hosts"; "Jehovah of the (Heavenly) Armies" (See 1 Samuel 17:45; Psalm 24:10.)
- *El Elyon*: "The Most High God"; "God Is the High One" (See Psalm 7:17; 47:2; 97:9.)
- *Jehovah Rohi*: "The Lord My Shepherd" (See Psalm 23:1; Psalm 80:1.)
- *Jehovah Tsidkenu*: "The Lord Our Righteousness" (See Jeremiah 23:6; 33:16.)
- *Jehovah Shammah*: "The Lord Is There" (See Ezekiel 48:35.)

In various lists of the names of God, you will find some variations in the spelling of the names and the specific descriptions used, but they are essentially the same.

There are a few things that stand out regarding the names of God. First, the Jewish community of Jesus's time would have been intimately familiar with God's names. They would have memorized them and called upon them when in need or celebration. They would have used those names when talking to others about God and His work, and there is something very beautiful about that.

Names in general were very important in Bible times because they denoted a particular quality or family trait. Sometimes names carried the hopes and dreams of the family, or they reflected an experience or a situation, and the names of God are no different. He delights when we use His names, when we know various facets of Him, and when we can find exactly what we need in Him.[41]

---

41. "Introduction," in "The Names of God in the Old Testament."

I (James) always saw my dad as my dad. But he was also a physician, and, while I was growing up, hearing others call him "doctor" was such a great reminder to me of who my dad was. He was my dad, yes, but he was also someone who helped and cared for others' health and bodies. This always gave me a better, more complete picture of my father, and it resulted in my having a more connected relationship with him because it allowed me to understand him and see him more fully. Similarly, as you meditate on God's names and what they mean, you will gain a more complete picture of who He is and be able to connect with Him more fully.

GOD'S NAMES AND THE LORD'S PRAYER

There are a few names of God that correspond wonderfully to the Lord's Prayer. When the disciples asked Jesus to show them how to pray, He famously gave them this incredible prayer. The Lord's Prayer was revolutionary for its day because it was simple and personal. At the time, God's followers were used to longer prayers that did not always touch on their personal lives. But Jesus's words in the Lord's Prayer removed the barrier between God and man. It was the first time that a rabbi (Jesus) demonstrated what talking directly to God could look like.

The Lord's Prayer has revolutionized my (Ronnie's) prayer life. I start my morning by praying Psalm 143 to help me get into the presence of God, and then I pray the Lord's Prayer. These are recited prayers, but there is power in them!

If you simply don't know what to pray, start with the prayer that Jesus provided for us:

> *This, then, is how you should pray: "Our Father in heaven, hallowed be your name, your kingdom come, your will be done, on earth as it is in heaven. Give us today our daily bread. And forgive us our debts, as we also have forgiven our debtors. And lead us not into temptation, but deliver us from the evil one."*
>
> (Matthew 6:9–13)

Other Bible translations, such as the King James Version, include this ending:

> For thine is the kingdom, and the power, and the glory, for ever. Amen. (Matthew 6:13 KJV)

So, let's look at a few powerful names of God and see how they correspond to the lines of the Lord's Prayer. Let this perspective reshape how you think about and use this ancient prayer, and let it also open your eyes to the blessings that await you when you begin to understand and incorporate the names of God into your prayer life.

El Shaddai

El Shaddai means "the Lord Almighty," "God Is the All-Powerful One," or "The All-Sufficient One."

Basically, this name is derived from the word "field," as in, "the fields produce abundance." It is also translated as "breast," or "the many-breasted One," which signifies nourishment and productiveness. In this sense, God is shown as the One who is more than enough—"He who is all-sufficient." When you see the name *El Shaddai*, God is saying, "I am more than enough to meet your needs in each situation."[42]

This name shows God's loving side and how He knows our needs and moves to meet them, much as a devoted mother cares for her children. "He is our sustainer."[43]

The first lines of the Lord's Prayer invoke *El Shaddai*. Though it is not specifically stated, the way Jesus approaches God is clearly from the position of His being almighty, all powerful, and all nurturing:

> Our Father in heaven, hallowed be your name, your kingdom come, your will be done, on earth as it is in heaven.
> (Matthew 6:9–10)

---

42. Hickey, *Names of God*, 37.
43. "El Shaddai (Lord God Almighty)," in "The Names of God in the Old Testament."

This opening address is all about who God is. He is exalted, high, mighty, and powerful. But it also touches on God's relationship with us—"*our Father*"—which is where the name *El Shaddai* comes in. God's kingdom is where we experience His presence. Asking for His kingdom to come is no different from asking for more of His presence in our lives. And as His will is done, we experience more of His blessings. So, claiming His lordship and calling on Him to bring His kingdom and will to earth is a direct ask that He step in and change our lives for His glory and blessing. This is the type of request a child would make of a parent. It is a request for nurturing and love.

Jehovah Nissi

Jehovah Nissi means "the Lord My Banner." This name can be translated to express the idea that God is our refuge or deliverer. In Exodus 17, the Israelites were battling the cruel Amalekites:

> In Moses' hands was the miracle-working rod of God that had brought terrible plagues upon the land of Egypt. This rod of God was more than a mere rod. It was the rod of God's mighty hand—the rod of *Elohim*!
>
> Moses was holding up the banner of God, which had brought victory to Israel. Moses was carrying a symbol of God's presence. As long as God's presence was established as the high standard, the Israelites prevailed in battle.
>
> When you hear the word *banner*, you probably picture a flag, but that is not necessarily what a banner was in Moses' day. It was often a bare pole with a bright and shining ornament that would glitter in the sun when held high in the air.
>
> The word for *banner* actually means "a glistening pole or ensign, a standard, or a miracle." The banner or "standard" represented God's cause. It was a symbol of His deliverance and mighty salvation that caused His people to be victors over their enemies.[44]

---

44. Hickey, *Names of God*, 90.

God is a warrior on our behalf, but, more than that, He is a victor. In the Lord's Prayer, we see *Jehovah Nissi* being indirectly referenced in Matthew 6:11:

> Give us today our daily bread.

Similar to His being like a banner on the battlefield and a victor in the battle, God provides us with all that we need to move forward with Him in life. This name is powerful for us as we follow Him because God meets our individual needs. He makes a way for us and for our victory when we move within His kingdom and His will.

We don't often think of ourselves as following God's banner, but that is one of the strongest visuals we can have of what it means to trust and follow Him wherever He leads. We trust Him for victory, we trust Him for provision, and we trust Him for safety.

Jesus already knows that our physical needs are important to the abundant life He promised us, but He wants us to come to Him *daily* for fellowship. That is such a key part of this verse—the daily call to partake and receive, to fellowship and delight in the Lord. And God will provide our bread. He will provide our victory. He will be our banner leading the way.

God could have provided Israel with a large quantity of manna to sustain them for years, but instead He chose to give them daily bread. He longs for connection. He longs to be in fellowship with us every step of the way.

Jehovah Shalom

This name means "the Lord Is Peace" or "the Lord Is My Peace and Wholeness." It occurs in Judges 6:23–24, where God encourages a fearful Gideon:

> The LORD said to him, "Peace! Do not be afraid. You are not going to die." So Gideon built an altar to the LORD there and called it The LORD Is Peace. To this day it stands in Ophrah of the Abiezrites.

God is the bringer and facilitator of peace, and this is the most powerful truth for our anxious minds. When we're feeling our fears, and when stressors get the better of us, we can call upon *Jehovah Shalom* and ask for His peace to overcome and push out the things that are getting to us.

But His peace isn't just for us—it's for everyone around us, too, which is why *Jehovah Shalom* comes to mind in reference to Matthew 6:12:

And forgive us our debts, as we also have forgiven our debtors.

If you're a Christian but have an unforgiving heart, you are going to have a lot of trouble experiencing forgiveness, because forgiving others and receiving forgiveness go together. An inability to forgive may indicate a bitter root within your heart, and this is something to take to your heavenly Father as you ask for His forgiveness and cleansing. Or perhaps you can't bring yourself to forgive someone due to the pain they have inflicted on you. This is where going to a trusted Christian counselor may be needed to help you work through this pain and to find the healing you need as you receive *Jehovah Shalom* as your Peace.

My (Ronnie's) dad was an overall handyman, and one of his jobs was to work as a plumber. This was back when the pipes were all made of lead, and you had to dig them out to physically see what the issue was. When I returned home for the summer while attending college, I would go help him on his jobs. We'd be digging, and finally he'd stop me and point to a small place where the pipes were joined together. Often, a small root, no bigger than my pinky finger, had grown in between the joints. When Dad opened up the pipe, it would frequently reveal a root ball that had completely blocked a portion of the pipe's interior. And since such pipes were usually connected to the sewer system, the blockage would have caused sewer water to back up into the house, making it nearly unlivable from the stench and sanitation issues.

Unforgiveness is like a small root that makes its way into your heart and life. It grows and grows, many times undetected, until it is a large root that has pushed everything else out and is completely blocking the path of all of the good things that God has for you. The writer of Hebrews tells us that a bitter root can "[grow] *up to cause trouble and defile many*" (Hebrews 12:15). Just one root of bitterness can ruin a person's entire life and negatively affect many more lives.

Jesus offers us forgiveness regardless of whether we do or don't forgive. But He also knows that when forgiveness is withheld by us and from us, it produces shame in us. And shame makes us want to separate ourselves from God and others. We should pause when we consider what Jesus said in the verses immediately following His model prayer for His disciples: *"For if you forgive other people when they sin against you, your heavenly Father will also forgive you. But if you do not forgive others their sins, your Father will not forgive your sins"* (Matthew 6:14–15).

From what I have read and heard from most scholars about this passage, the implication is that if we lack an attitude of forgiveness for others, we will not be able to experience God's forgiveness in our own lives. But could it be that much of the anxiety and even depression we experience is due to the burden of the sins we carry when we have not forgiven others, along with the burden we carry when we do not feel God has forgiven us—when He actually has? This is like a man who continues to sit in a jail cell even though he has been told by the prison authorities that he is free, and the door to his cell has been unlocked. The *fact* of what God has done for us through the person of Jesus is what is imperative to the truth, but what we *claim* is true for us affects what we feel—whether peace from God or shame from Satan.

Shame tells us that we aren't good enough to be forgiven and to receive what God offers. But God tells us that we can have peace. We can change our thinking, our patterns, and our habits. We are not doomed for *anything*. Life is about forgiveness, and forgiveness is about second chances.

Shame will tell you that you can't forgive or that you can't receive forgiveness. It will tell you that you aren't worthy of any of it. But the God of peace, *Jehovah Shalom*, quiets those criticisms and treats those wounds. He offers freedom from bitterness, resentment, anger, and so much more. He brings peace because He *is* peace.

El Elyon

El Elyon means "the Most High God" or "God Is the High One."

El Elyon comes from the root word *alah*, meaning "to go up, ascend, climb, or exalt." It is a name that says there is no existing thing that is higher than the Most High God. He is the possessor of heaven, earth, and everything in them. His name is so high, so exalted, and so marvelous that there is no other name to compare with His name.[45]

This name reminds us of how big God is and how everything truly is in His hand. Nothing is outside His control or power. But, in tandem with God's bigness, He also wants personal fellowship with us.

Think of it! The God of the universe, who is eternal and beyond time, who created everything we know and see and love in the natural world, deeply wants a relationship and fellowship with each of us. There is nothing that would ever surprise Him, no problem that would be beyond His capacity to solve. His greatness is impossible to comprehend, and yet He loves you. He loves us. And He desires to be in fellowship with us.

If God can manage the universe, He can certainly protect us. Matthew 6:13 of the Lord's Prayer reads:

And lead us not into temptation, but deliver us from the evil one.

The Lord sent us an Advocate—the Holy Spirit—to be with us and to help us forever. (See, for example, John 15:26.) This Advocate,

---

45. Hickey, *Names of God*, 150.

the Spirit of Truth, lives within us, helping us and guiding us. We tend to live as though this isn't a big deal, when, in reality, it's miraculous—the God of the universe is within us! This is more than the Israelites of the Old Testament ever hoped for: God and man, existing together.

How would your life be different if you lived with an awareness that the almighty God is within you, ready to help you? He is present to bring you out of temptation and to point you toward Christ so that you can experience all of His blessings.

We forget this. We think that we have to do life on our own, that we are responsible for getting it all right. But *El Elyon* is with us, even now, delivering us out of darkness and into light.

Jehovah Rapha

Jehovah Rapha, "the Lord Who Heals You" or "the Lord My Health," is a picture of God as a physician, healing the spiritual, emotional, and physical needs of His people.[46] It can be hard to know how to pray for someone who is ill, yet Philippians 4:6 tells us to go to God *"in every situation,"* and this would include times when we need healing (especially when we are anxious about it!).

This does not mean that God is a genie in a bottle, healing us as soon as we ask. We know of at least two people in the Bible who were witnesses to Christ (Paul and Timothy), and yet both had chronic problems that God chose not to heal.

In chapter 1, we talked briefly about Paul's *"thorn in [the] flesh"* (2 Corinthians 12:7). The nature of this *"thorn"* is not clear, but we do know that it was *"a messenger of Satan"* that was sent to torment him. (See 2 Corinthians 12:7.) Paul prayed three times that God would remove the thorn, and God chose not to. Yet, the Lord spoke to Paul and said, *"My grace is sufficient for you, for my power is made perfect in*

---

46. "Jehovah Rapha (The Lord Who Heals)," in "The Names of God in the Old Testament."

weakness" (verse 9). Paul learned to delight in his weaknesses, finding that when he struggled, God gave him strength. (See verse 9.)

In 1 Timothy 5:23, Paul told Timothy to use a little wine because of his frequent stomach illnesses. So we know that Timothy struggled with a stomach ailment and managed it with medication. Although we don't know the background to this and whether Timothy and Paul had prayed for Timothy's healing, it would seem likely that they did, so this appears to be another example where God chose not to heal in a direct way.

When it comes to physical healing, there are times when *Jehovah Rapha* chooses to fully heal. There are times when He offers partial healing. And there are times when we must simply wait. God doesn't always choose to heal like we want Him to, but, more than anything, *Jehovah Rapha* is interested in our spiritual healing and spiritual health. Yes, He cares deeply about our mental, emotional, and physical health, but we also live in a broken world. Ultimate healing will not come until God creates the new heavens and new earth, when everything broken will be made right. (See Revelation 21:1–5.)

Until then, we pray and trust. We pray to *Jehovah Rapha* for physical, mental, and spiritual health, knowing that full healing will come with Jesus's return. We are reminded of this in the closing of the Lord's Prayer:

> *For thine is the kingdom, and the power, and the glory, for ever. Amen.* (Matthew 6:13 KJV)

God's perspective is so different from our own. He sees what we cannot see: the intricacies of the world around us. I think of how easy it is for us to look around and see something that someone else has that appears to be so much better than what we currently have. For example, it's easy to think, "I want *that* [job, opportunity, position, relationship, or possession]." But God sees the snakes hiding in the green grass, the stumbling blocks along the seemingly easy path. He knows our hearts, and just because something looks good doesn't mean it is—or that it is right for us or the best thing for us at this time. Or, we may experience the difficult parts of our journey in order to help someone else on the hard part of their journey. Following *Jehovah Rapha* means trusting His heart and hand, trusting the Shepherd.

Knowing that full healing is not always what God has for us, how might that change your perspective, your heart, your posture? How might that change your algorithm? This earthly life is but the blink of an eye compared to eternity spent in wholeness, healing, and freedom with our Lord, and so we give glory to our King in the here and now, no matter what our circumstances. We pray for healing, but we do so with open hands, knowing that God sees the big picture, and His peace is more than enough to cover us.

Jehovah Rohi

We touched on God being our Shepherd, and this is the name that reflects that quality: *Jehovah Rohi*, "the Lord My Shepherd." God takes care of His sheep, protecting them and leading them. What's really poignant about this quality is that shepherds know their sheep on an individual level. They know their personalities, their quirks. They know their tendencies and their trouble spots.

A beautiful translation of *rohi* is "companion or friend." This expresses the idea of intimacy and sharing life and food. Jesus is our great Shepherd, and we are intimate with Him. The Bible says that we are joint heirs with Him (see Romans 8:17); we are to share in His life and identify completely with Him. Exodus 33:11 spoke of a *rohi* relationship between the Lord and Moses: "*The* LORD *spake unto Moses face to face, as a man speaketh unto his friend.*"[47]

---

47. Hickey, *The Names of God*, 132–133.

Thinking about God as our Shepherd reminds us of how He fully knows and sees us, how He loves us, and how He wants to be our Friend and Confidant.[48]

In Jesus, God lowered Himself to our level—He became human and suffered and died as a human. He did all this so that we could be in relationship with Him, so that He could fully know us and we could know Him, and so that He could shepherd us.

When we look at the Lord's Prayer as a whole, we see *Jehovah Rohi*, the caring Shepherd who provides for His sheep, protects them, and leads them toward the kingdom. This is the God we serve, and this is the God who longs to free you from the stress and anxiety that overtakes you.

EVERY GOOD THING

Praying the names of God can revolutionize your prayer life—but remember that it doesn't always mean you'll get what you ask for. In fact, most of the time, what we think we want is not what we need! In Matthew 7, Jesus said:

> *Which of you, if your son asks for bread, will give him a stone? Or if he asks for a fish, will give him a snake? If you, then, though you are evil, know how to give good gifts to your children, how much more will your Father in heaven give good gifts to those who ask him!* (Matthew 7:9–11)

The biggest thing that I (Ronnie) struggle with in this verse is the word *"good."* Many times, we have a different perspective from God on what a "good" gift should be. Sometimes we get tripped up on the things of this world, thinking that money or success or popularity is a "good" gift. Other times, the "good" gifts that we want really are in line with the goodness of God! We ask for healing from a particular disease or the restoration of a particular relationship or freedom from a particular sinful habit—but even praying for the right things

---

48. "Jehovah-Raah (The Lord My Shepherd)," in "The Names of God in the Old Testament."

does not guarantee that God will "deliver," especially in our preferred timing.

We must learn to trust God's definition of good (specifically with regard to our situation) more than our own.

I have gotten myself into so much trouble trying to define what is good. When Anne and I moved to Hattiesburg after my residency, we decided to buy a home that would not put our family in a financial strain. So, we bought a small but comfortable house. After three years, we found ourselves with three children, and suddenly that small but comfortable home was no longer very comfortable! We had previously purchased land in the country and were praying for God's direction about building our "forever" home. We had plans drawn up and were talking to a builder when our church entered a building project and asked for three-year pledges to fund the project. We prayed and could not get away from the direction God was taking us to put a hold on our new home and commit that money to the church-building project instead. We really thought our home was a good idea, but it ended up not being the right idea for that time in our lives. After another three years, we started the home-building project again. In the meantime, a builder had joined our Sunday school class at church, and when we told him of our plans, he said he could build us twice the house for the same amount of money—and he did! Doing God's will may not always result in a double blessing, but that time it did.

There are many aspects of "good," but God's good is always the best.

What if we approached life truly believing that God—with all of His names, qualities, and abilities—was with us every step of the way? What if we fully believed that He had our backs and that His way was best because He sees and knows all? What if we set down our own agendas, fears, insecurities, and stressors and received all of the facets of God, knowing and believing that He is for us?

How would that define your algorithm? How would that affect your anxiety?

As Paul closed his letter to the Philippians, he wanted them to realize the fruits of a life in Jesus, and why it's so worthwhile to take fellowship with Christ seriously. When we talk to God, we draw closer to Him. And when we are closer to Him, His peace—along with all of His other attributes and blessings—is available to us in the gentlest way.

Jesus is calling us to a higher place where we are able to function fully, where anxiety no longer hinders our love and service toward God and others. This isn't about "being so heavenly minded that we aren't any earthly good." It's about realizing that we are strangers in a strange land, and we aren't home yet.

This life is hard. There will be stress and fear and anxiety. But there can also be much peace and comfort from our Healer, our Shepherd, our Lord Almighty.

◇ ◇ ◇

WELLNESS EXERCISE: PRAY THE NAMES OF GOD

Go to the list of names of God in chapter 21 and review each name and its meaning. Next, write down each name and match it to an area of your life where you need God to help you in that way. For example, for *Jehovah Rapha*, write down something in your life that needs healing. It might be physical, mental, spiritual, or relational healing. Then, go through the names one by one again as you pray, and ask God to reveal Himself to you through these qualities, praising Him for His many attributes. Keep track of how God moves in your life.

Remember, God knows all. Even if He does not "fix" your need in the way you thought He would, He *will* be faithful to walk with you in life if you have the eyes to see Him and the ears to hear Him.

22

THE SECRET OF CONTENTMENT

The Bible says that a defining mark of Christians is the way that we love. (See John 13:35.) While that is absolutely true, we think it's also true—especially today, in America's anxiety-filled society—that those of us who are Christians should be able to be identified by our *contentment*.

In a culture that chases after the next job promotion, the next opportunity, the next home, the next gadget, the next relationship, we have an opportunity to show a different way of life—a life that is rooted in contentment and fulfillment no matter what.

We lose our contentment when we start to worry too much, and we start to worry too much when our concern for others or for various situations becomes magnified. Paul praised the Philippians for their "renewed concern" for him. (See Philippians 4:10.) It was *good* that they were concerned and praying and moving on his behalf. So, let it be clear: there is nothing wrong with being concerned for others or even for ourselves. The problem comes when our concern drives us to anxiety. When that happens, the relationship or issue that we are concerned about ends up taking too much ownership of our lives. We feel more responsibility for the outcome than we should, and we move from a healthy concern into an anxiety-based fear. We move from prayer and petitioning and stepping out confidently to taking action (intervening) when the Lord directs to full-blown panic attacks and fear-ridden paralysis.

Being content means being fulfilled and at peace regardless of what you or those around you are facing. It means rejoicing even when money is tight or your career takes a bad turn. It means praying earnestly for God to move while also trusting in His promises.

Contentment is the key to a joyful and peaceful life. This is a reality that the scientific world recognizes. Neuroscientist and podcaster Dr. Andrew Huberman, along with his guest, Dr. Paul Conti, discussed in a September 6, 2023, podcast that one way we may describe someone who is in a state of well-being is that they have "peace, contentment, and delight."[49] In other words, they believe that someone who is content also has wellness. Someone who is at peace has wellness. Someone who delights in life has wellness.

The dictionary defines *contented* as "feeling or showing satisfaction with one's possessions, status, or situation,"[50] but, for so many of us, satisfaction, peace, and contentment feel impossible because we're so worried about tomorrow. We're worried about things not going the way we want them to go and people not doing what we want them to do.

We worry, and we wait for things to change. But contentment doesn't just happen to you. It's not something you are handed once you make a certain amount of money or buy the right car or have your name on a Times Square advertisement.

Contentment can be learned. It can be practiced. And, ultimately, it comes from God.

THE SECRET

> *I am not saying this because I am in need, for I have learned to be content whatever the circumstances.* (Philippians 4:11)

---

49. Andrew Huberman and Dr. Paul Conti, "How to Understand and Assess Your Mental Health," Huberman Lab Guest Series, 2:21:33, https://youtu.be/tLRCS48Ens4.

50. *Merriam-Webster.com Dictionary*, s.v. "contented," accessed October 22, 2024, https://www.merriam-webster.com/dictionary/contented.

In this passage, Paul implies that, at one point in his life, he wasn't content. And if contentment is something Paul struggled with, certainly it's something that we might struggle with as well. But struggling with contentment doesn't have to be a permanent state. We can move toward growth in that area, much as we strive to move toward growth in all areas of life.

Once more, most people think that success or financial security or physical health or right relationships is the key to contentment. But Paul says that the key is in our Lord, who gives us the strength we need to learn contentment:

> *I know what it is to be in need, and I know what it is to have plenty. I have learned the secret of being content in any and every situation, whether well fed or hungry, whether living in plenty or in want. I can do all this through him who gives me strength.*
> (Philippians 4:12–13)

Why does Paul call what he has learned about contentment a *"secret"*? We believe that he used this word because the answer is so different from what most people imagine. Rather than contentment being linked to situations or possessions or people, the real source and secret of contentment is that, through Christ—who never changes and who has promised never to leave us as He provides the abundant life He promised—we can rise above the ever-changing, ever-unpredictable aspects of life. (See, for example, Matthew 28:20; Hebrews 13:8.)

We can do this—we can learn to be content because of Christ, who provides us with peace and joy and fulfillment. Simply telling ourselves to be content is not going to do it. Even looking at everything God has given us isn't going to do it. In fact, looking at those things may make us more anxious as we realize that we *should* be content yet aren't.

Not only is God the One who provides contentment, but He is also the One who reveals to us the things that lead toward contentment, such as the fruit of the Spirit that we read about in Galatians 5.

So, when we say that contentment is learned, we mean that we can't produce contentment on our own. But we can take steps to welcome it as we embrace a life with Christ and allow Him to do much of the heavy lifting. As we abide in Him, as we develop an ever-deepening relationship with Him, He produces in us the contentment that leads to peace that we really cannot explain, that *"transcends all understanding"* (Philippians 4:7). Just like fruit that "abides" on the vine, as we "hang in there" with Christ, and as His Spirit flows into us, and we ripen in Him, we become more mature. We won't be fully ripe or perfect until we see Jesus face-to-face, but we can move toward that maturity every day as we allow Him to produce it in us.

A key verse for me (Ronnie) is Psalm 37:4, which reads, *"Take delight in the* LORD, *and he will give you the desires of your heart."* In the past, I thought this meant that God would give us what we wanted, but I now believe it means much more than that. If you delight in your desires (the things you want), then your contentment will be limited to whether or not those things happen. But if you delight in God, your contentment will be found purely in Him—and that's when He will surprise you by giving you various desires of your heart!

This key to contentment isn't merely a secret; it's a true miracle. And that is what people need to see—a contentment that rises above anything the world can offer. A contentment that the world is desperately seeking.

Contentment that comes from Christ wards off anxiety. We see an example of this in 2 Corinthians 8:1–5, where Paul states that the Macedonian churches had experienced *"a very severe trial."* Remarkably, instead of this situation causing them stress and anxiety, it produced in them *"overflowing joy."* This joy and their *"extreme poverty"* resulted in *"rich generosity."* (See verse 2.)

This scenario is something that just doesn't make sense to those of us in the midst of anxiety and stress. Suffering should not bring joy. The extreme poverty that Paul wrote about should not bring about generosity. But that is exactly what these churches experienced.

Despite what was probably a life-threatening situation, they had incredible joy and generosity.

The churches in Macedonia had found *the secret*. They had given themselves completely over to Christ. It didn't matter what happened to them or how much they were struggling. All that mattered was Him.

In Romans 12:1, Paul encourages, *"Therefore, I urge you, brothers and sisters, in view of God's mercy, to offer your bodies as a living sacrifice."* When we give ourselves to God, something changes. Joy replaces our anguish. Contentment replaces our fear and need for control.

OUR ULTIMATE SOURCE OF HOPE

And my God will meet all your needs according to the riches of his glory in Christ Jesus. To our God and Father be glory for ever and ever. Amen. (Philippians 4:19–20)

Do you believe that God will meet all of your needs? Do you believe that He will come through for you? Do these words from Philippians ring true to you, or are you holding on to doubt? Do you think that God doesn't show up for you the way He shows up for others? Or maybe you doubt His plan, afraid that if you let go control of your life, He will take you somewhere you don't want to go.

Maybe you trust yourself more than you trust Him?

God operates in a way that we can't even fathom. The things that we think are important are but a tiny part of a much bigger, more beautiful plan. Our view is so narrow, so limited, and all He wants us to do is to sit back and watch Him work.

This isn't about getting what we want. God meets our needs—He doesn't always meet our wants. This is about the promise of goodness being given to us when we seek the kingdom of God. (See Matthew 6:33.) Everything God gives is good. Everything He gives is needed. Everything He provides is for our benefit and the benefit of others. As we've said previously, He's not a genie in a bottle that you can call upon for three wishes. He is a loving Father who gives to His children and provides for their journeys.

PUTTING IT ALL TOGETHER

Which part of this book most spoke to you and the specific anxiety you are dealing with? Was it the Two Steps Back method, where you saw you could calm your thoughts and develop new clarity about your situation? Was it a particular wellness quality from Philippians 4:8 that you began to focus on and realized it was helping to dispel your fears? Was it a specific name of God that enabled you to hand your worries over to Him to take care of? Maybe it was an understanding of your need for supportive relationships in your life. Or perhaps it was the simple breathing exercise, which enabled your body to let go of some of your stress.

We believe that all these elements, as well as the other principles and wellness exercises we have presented in this book, will make a significant difference in your life as you regularly put them into practice. Start with those areas that have especially helped to show you there is a way through your stress, anxiety, and fear to a life of joy and peace. Then, as you take the time to build your personalized algorithm and chart your Thought Record, commit to applying these helps each day as you experience recurring anxiety or whenever you need a mindset of peace.

Remember, it will take time and hard work to form new habits and leave behind old tendencies that keep you in anxiety and stress. But it is well worth it!

This is our prayer for you on your journey toward wellness:

> The LORD bless you
> and keep you;
> the LORD make his face shine on you
> and be gracious to you;
> the LORD turn his face toward you
> and give you peace.   (Numbers 6:24–26)

AN INVITATION

As you've read this book, maybe you've wondered if you have the same type of relationship with Jesus that we (James and Ronnie) describe. Maybe you are aware that you don't have a relationship with Jesus, but you would like to know Him. Initiating or deepening a relationship with Jesus is not difficult, but it is a significant commitment. Let us explain.

The Bible is clear that Jesus came and sacrificed Himself for us all so that we could be restored to God, our heavenly Father. (See John 3:16–17.) Jesus came to save the world. In order to be one of His followers, there are a few things you have to truly believe and arrange your life around:

- Jesus is God's Son—He is both fully God and fully man. You do not have to completely understand how this is possible. Believing is about having faith and trusting God even when you can't understand His ways.
- Jesus died and was buried, and God raised Him from the dead.
- Jesus died in your place, receiving the penalty for your sins.

The Bible tells us that *"all have sinned and fall short of the glory of God"* (Romans 3:23), and that the penalty for sin is death. (See Romans 6:23.) Death is a consequence of sin. That may seem harsh, but it goes all the way back to the garden of Eden in the book of Genesis, where God said that He had to remove the first human beings, Adam and Eve, from the garden after they went against His warning and ate of the Tree of Knowledge of Good and Evil. There was another tree in the garden: the Tree of (eternal) Life. God had to remove Adam and Eve because He did not want them to eat of the Tree of Life and be stuck forever in a sinful state. (See Genesis 3:22–23.) So, He put a plan in motion to restore any human who would trust Him and His process of salvation. This process centered on the person of Jesus Christ. After expressing that the penalty for sin is death, Romans 6:23 goes on to say, *"But the gift of God is eternal life in Christ Jesus our Lord."*

You must believe in your heart that Jesus paid your debt, that He took your place and was guilty in your stead. This means that you need to accept the forgiveness of your sin that He offers. This is called grace—receiving what you don't deserve (none of us does).

You can never "earn" heaven. The only way to be forgiven, be restored to the Father, and receive eternal life is through Jesus's sacrifice for you. When you accept His sacrifice, it is normal to feel grateful to Him and to feel a desire to praise and worship God because He made a way for you to return to Him. He put this way into motion thousands of years ago—really, before time began. (See Revelation 13:8.)

This is just the beginning of your new life. Once you understand who Jesus is and what He has done for you, and you choose to follow Him with your whole heart, you will start to change the way you think and live because He has asked you to and because you now have a new nature in Jesus. In this book, we have talked about practicing the "spiritual disciplines." These include reading your Bible (hopefully daily) so that you can learn more and more about who God is; fellowshipping with other believers, which is typically done by joining a church and attending regularly; praying (a fancy word for "talking to God"); and committing to following God's way over your way. You "die to yourself" and say that, from now on, you are going to do your best to make Jesus the center of your life. (See, for example, Galatians 2:20.)

That's it—we (James and Ronnie) have just unpacked the gospel message, the "good news," for you. Your purpose now is to practice living it out for the rest of your life. The best news is that God did not leave that part up to us either. He sent Jesus to live the sinless life we couldn't live and to pay the penalty of death that we couldn't pay. He then sent us His Holy Spirit to help us live the life He has called us to live. (See, for example, John 14:25–26.) What good news—what fabulous news! The Bible tells us that God is faithful to teach us and to walk with us through life, enabling us to grow so that we will become more and more like Jesus. Our hope is that everyone would know Him and what it means to be a child of God. (See John 1:12.)

As we wrote at the beginning of this book, our role in *The Anxiety Algorithm* is to usher you into an awareness of the presence of almighty God—a place of peace and joy where wellness occurs.

◇ ◇ ◇

EXAMPLES OF PERSONALIZING THE ANXIETY ALGORITHM

The algorithm is meant to be deeply personal. There really is no right or wrong way to create it, although, for it to be most effective, it is important for you to seek Christ and listen to the Spirit as you do so. To help show the range of ways in which the algorithm may be used, we asked a few friends to share their experiences. You will see that an algorithm can incorporate both words and pictures. We hope that these examples spark ideas and give you the freedom to craft an algorithm that speaks directly to you.

AMANDA

I love worshipping God through song. A few years ago, I decided to implement daily praise and worship into my routine. I committed to do this for a month. Every day, I'd put on my favorite worship playlist and sing along while making dinner or going about my day. The results were astounding. By the end of the month, I felt more joyful than I'd ever felt in my life—and this was in spite of very, very painful family problems that were doing major damage and tearing the family apart.

I simply could not believe that singing songs to God had such a direct and noticeable impact on my mood and outlook!

Knowing this, when I formed my algorithm, I did so with music in mind. I have a very specific playlist that I use to recenter my thoughts and turn my focus to God. I sing about who God is, the promises He has made, and the amazing truth that He is able to do anything.

Singing these songs when I feel a downward spiral has helped to soften my heart against people who have hurt me. It has routinely pulled me out of states of hopelessness and infused me with faith and trust. And it has set my sights on what really matters: a relationship with God and His Spirit.

KA

(Ka was a class member who shared with us their main focal points for each of the algorithm categories, plus the verses that they used:)

True: God's Word and Promise

"Do not fear, for I am with you; do not be afraid, for I am your God. I will strengthen you; I will help you; I will hold on to you with my righteous right hand" (Isaiah 41:10).

Noble: Christ Died on the Cross for Me

I have been redeemed from the curse of the law because Jesus was made a curse for me (on the cross). (Galatians 3:13)

Right: Live Bringing Glory to God's Kingdom

Let your light so shine among men that they may see your good deeds and give glory to your Father in heaven. (Matthew 5:16)

Pure: God's Peace

This day I choose to let the peace of God rule in my heart. I refuse to worry about anything. (Colossians 3:15)

Lovely: God's Creation

God saw all that He made, and it was very good. (Genesis 1:1–31)

Admirable: God's Grace

"*For all have sinned and fall short of the glory of God, and all are justified freely by his grace through the redemption that came by Christ Jesus*" (Romans 3:23–24).

Excellent: God's Blessings

I praise You, Father, that the blessing of Abraham belongs to me. I am blessed in every way. (Deuteronomy 28:1–14)

Praiseworthy: God!!!

"*For he will command his angels concerning you to guard you in all your ways*" (Psalm 91:11).

CHRIS

(Chris really became invested in the algorithm, and he put together this flowchart to help him stay focused.)

CHRISTOPHER CREECH'S ANXIETY ALGORITHM
Inspired by Philippians 4:8

"*Finally, brothers and sisters, whatever is true, whatever is noble, whatever is right, whatever is pure, whatever is lovely, whatever is admirable—if anything is excellent or praiseworthy—think about such things.*"

TRUTH IN ANXIETY

"*Little children, let us not love in word or talk but in deed and truth.*"
—1 John 3:18

I try to bring truth and grace when sharing my everyday truth by not only speaking truth but showing truth.

My "truth" is I AM ALIVE!! I don't think I'm worthy of my life but Jesus does, and that TRUTH calms me and keeps my head held high.

CHRISTOPHER CREECH'S ANXIETY ALGORITHM
Inspired by Philippians 4:8

NOBLE IN ANXIETY

"But he who is noble plans noble things, and on noble things he stands."
—Isaiah 32:8

An act or deed for others for the betterment of them and/or the greater "them."

My "noble" act is recognizing that sometimes I need to step aside and trust that there are others who are better at accomplishing a certain task/act.

RIGHT IN ANXIETY

"The father of the righteous will greatly rejoice; he who fathers a wise son will be glad in him."
—Proverbs 23:24

One who stays on the path even when surrounded by negativity.

I think of my son as "right" or "righteous." He is as close as any human I know with the kindest heart and soul, and it calms my anxiety…even if he is the one who caused my anxiety…lol.

PURE IN ANXIETY

"Let no one despise you for your youth, but set the believers an example in speech, in conduct, in love, in faith, in purity."
—1 Timothy 4:12

My son's inexperienced and faithful heart. Let it never change.

My son has grounded me in his goodness, and I cherish the gift of him from God every day.

CHRISTOPHER CREECH'S ANXIETY ALGORITHM
Inspired by Philippians 4:8

LOVELY IN ANXIETY

"Hallelujah! How good it is to sing to our God, for praise is pleasant and lovely.... He heals the brokenhearted and binds up their wounds."
—Psalm 147:1, 3

Lovely translated from Greek is *prosphilēs* (pros-fee-lace'), meaning acceptable and pleasing.

My roses are my piece of God's acceptable and pleasing part of heaven here on earth. When I'm low, I look at my roses and pray a prayer of thankfulness.

ADMIRABLE IN ANXIETY

*"And I prayed to the L*ORD*, 'O Lord G*OD*, do not destroy your people and your heritage, whom you have redeemed through your greatness, whom you have brought out of Egypt with a mighty hand. Remember your servants, Abraham, Isaac, and Jacob. Do not regard the stubbornness of this people, or their wickedness or their sin.'"*
—Deuteronomy 9:26–27

I think of Moses. He should be bitter and forsake the people for their weakness and losing faith so quickly, but he doesn't and prostrates himself before the Lord and prays and pleads for their lives. I can't think of many who are more admirable than Moses, and I will keep trying to be like Moses even when I'm anxious.

EXCELLENT OR PRAISEWORTHY IN ANXIETY

*"I love you, O L*ORD*, my strength. The L*ORD *is my rock and my fortress and my deliverer, my God, my rock, in whom I take refuge, my shield, and the horn of my salvation, my stronghold. I call upon the L*ORD*, who is worthy to be praised, and I am saved from my enemies."*
—Psalm 18:1–3

God's love and forgiveness, especially for me and my many flaws. I am not worthy but praise Him that He thinks I am.

ACKNOWLEDGMENTS

To our church family at Temple Baptist, who provide great fellowship, encouragement, and a place to try out our material before it is put into print.

To our friends who are so encouraging and hold us accountable in our walk.

To our friends at JourneyWise, who launched us and gave us great ideas and encouragement.

To Amanda Luedeke, who helped this course look like a book. What a miracle worker!

To Lois Puglisi at Whitaker House, who brought additional clarity, put on the polish, and made it shine.

To all the folks at Whitaker House for their encouragement and spiritual support.

ABOUT THE AUTHORS

JAMES KENT, PSYD, has over ten years of experience as a psychotherapist in clinical practice, working with teenagers, adults, couples, and families with a variety of mental health needs and concerns. He currently serves as the director of Twelve:Thirty, a not-for-profit ministry (based on Mark 12:30) seeking to provide education and resources for individuals and churches in the areas of wellness and mental health. He is particularly interested in the intersection of Christian faith and psychology and in helping others connect with Jesus Christ. James earned his doctoral degree in clinical psychology from Wheaton College. He is happily married to his wife, Jessica, and they share four wonderful children together. The family lives in Hattiesburg, Mississippi.

RONNIE KENT, MD, recently retired after a forty-one-year practice as a board-certified pediatrician and behavioral health specialist in Hattiesburg, Mississippi. He founded Connections Clinic and spent twenty-five years focused on treating children and adolescents with problems at school and related disorders, primarily

ADHD, learning disabilities, behavioral issues, anxiety, and depression. Ronnie is a graduate of the University of Mississippi (UM) and the UM School of Medicine. He is currently the codirector of Twelve:Thirty, a not-for-profit ministry (based on Mark 12:30) seeking to provide education and resources for individuals and churches in the areas of wellness and mental health. He and his wife, Anne, have been married for forty-five years and have three adult children and ten grandchildren. Ronnie has been teaching Bible classes in churches for decades, and his multiple hobbies include woodworking, gardening, and beekeeping, but especially spending time with his wonderful family.

For more information about Twelve:Thirty ministry, please visit https://1230ministry.com/.